HOW TO THRIVE AS A NEWLY QUALIFIED NURSE

This book is dedicated to every newly qualified nurse choosing to represent our noble profession, and its contents have been informed by their experiences and feedback.

You are the backbone of the NHS and deserve respect, care and structured support throughout your journey ahead.

HOW TO THRIVE AS A NEWLY QUALIFIED NURSE

CAROL FORDE-JOHNSTON

RGN, BSc Hons, PGDip, RNT, MSc

Lecturer Practitioner, Oxford Brookes University and
Oxford University Hospitals NHS Foundation Trust

Lantern

ISBN 9781908625519

First published in 2019 by Lantern Publishing Ltd

Lantern Publishing Ltd, The Old Hayloft, Vantage Business Park, Bloxham Rd, Banbury OX16 9UX, UK

www.lanternpublishing.com

British Library Cataloguing in Publication Data
A catalogue record for this book is available from the British Library

The authors and publisher have made every attempt to ensure the content of this book is up to date and accurate. However, healthcare knowledge and information is changing all the time so the reader is advised to double-check any information in this text on drug usage, treatment procedures, the use of equipment, etc. to confirm that it complies with the latest safety recommendations, standards of practice and legislation, as well as local Trust policies and procedures. Students are advised to check with their tutor and/or mentor before carrying out any of the procedures in this textbook.

Use the free Learning Diary app from FourteenFish to record your notes and reflection as you read this book.

www.fourteenfish.com/app

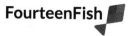

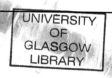
Typeset by Medlar Publishing Solutions Pvt Ltd, India

Cover design by AM Design

Printed in the UK

Last digit is the print number: 10 9 8 7 6 5 4

Distributed by NBN International, 10 Thornbury Rd, Plymouth, PL6 7PP, UK

CONTENTS

ABOUT THE AUTHOR

Carol Forde-Johnston (RGN, BSc Hons, PGDip, RNT and MSc) is a lecturer practitioner, a joint appointment between Oxford Brookes University and Oxford University Hospitals NHS Foundation Trust. She qualified as a registered nurse in 1989 at Coventry School of Nursing and went on to specialise in neurosciences, working her way up to G grade nursing sister. Carol has worked for 20 years in her ideal job as a lecturer practitioner, enabling her to integrate research, education and clinical practice into her role. She has published numerous articles relating to education and practice development in UK and European nursing and medical journals.

Carol leads a third year nursing module at Oxford Brookes University and supports newly qualified nurses and apprentices as part of her hospital trust role. In 2015, as part of a hospital trust steering group, she created and evaluated a *three-tiered curriculum Foundation Preceptorship programme* for all newly qualified nurses within the Oxford University Hospitals NHS Foundation Trust. The programme integrated skills development, theoretical study days and clinical supervision using action learning sets.

Carol has also been involved in several patient improvement initiatives and collaborated with Oxford University on a staff-led quality improvement project to prevent inpatient hospital falls. She is currently in her third year at the University of Southampton studying for a PhD in health sciences and plans to conduct an observational study examining nurse–patient interactions at the bedside in hospital wards that use a scripted approach during intentional rounding. Carol is passionate about developing and supporting newly qualified nurses and student nurses to improve their confidence when they qualify.

PREFACE

This book has grown from 20 years of supporting pre-registration nursing students and newly qualified nurses in my role as a lecturer practitioner, and 30 years working in clinical practice. It provides a survival manual full of tips to help you thrive during your training and when you qualify. You may refer to its contents frequently when writing assignments or come back to it when experiencing challenging issues in practice, as key topics are based on the reality experienced by newly qualified nurses.

This book aims to help:

- pre-registration student nurses, as a simple guide to direct their skill development during their training and their first year qualified
- university lecturers and clinical educators teaching nurses, who can use the boxes, tables and practical advice to educate students or newly qualified nurses
- nursing associate nurses planning to develop their skills further to become a registered nurse
- nurses returning to practice after a career break needing to increase their knowledge of current practices
- non-UK trained nurses planning to work in the UK, to increase their knowledge of UK nursing practice and standards.

Student nurses must navigate complex modular degree programmes whilst completing clinical competencies to develop their practical skills, amid challenging health care environments. There is a need for closer partnership between UK health care institutions that support clinical placements and sign-off of competencies, and universities that provide theory to underpin clinical practice and the assessment of student skills during laboratory simulations. The vocational, theoretical and professional aspects of nursing are interdependent, and require direct collaboration between these independent institutions, such as joint appointments to clinical education posts.

Newly qualified nurses deserve structured support on qualification from expert clinical role models, and this support should be assured and not dependent on where they choose to work in the UK. New starter nurses and students are bombarded with standards and policies that they must adhere to. Sometimes they just need a gentle hand guiding them through this complexity, and this book sets out to provide practical guidance as an antidote to these challenges.

Each chapter begins with a case example from newly qualified nurses, identifying areas where they required additional support, to place chapters in context. Important areas are covered, such as how to choose your first post, how to structure your learning during your first year qualified, what you need to know about safe staffing, how to prioritise and delegate care, how to assess mental capacity, what to do if an individual declines care, and how to escalate or report an incident. Not every aspect of specialist care can be covered, but the practical guidance offered will help to structure your learning and give you insights into the support you can access.

Since the 1980s I have heard so many buzzwords and NHS jargon, reflecting what is in vogue at the time, usually influenced by the latest management guru. We cannot, however, provide '*innovative*', '*evidence-based health care*' and '*assure positive patient clinical outcomes*', or '*maintain quality standards*' without highly trained nurses who are supported to thrive when they qualify by expert role models and post-registration development.

Our future nursing workforce relies on investment in newly qualified nurses' education and the development of nursing career pathways to retain staff. It is not just about developing '*resilience*' and the ability of individuals to cope with incessant pressure, whilst not maintaining staffing levels conducive to quality care. Yes, nurses need to take responsibility for their learning and development following qualification, but governments should be accountable for sustaining safe nurse staffing levels throughout the NHS by providing enough nurse training places. Health care employers should provide structured clinical education on qualification, to give every new starter the chance to thrive and reach their full potential.

The final chapter in this book focuses on the importance of nursing research in the future. I hope more nurses are inspired to conduct research examining what nurses do, the influence of staffing ratios on nurse–patient interactions, how long it takes to do what we do properly, and how that aligns with patient dependency and staffing levels. Such research can only empower our profession and influence positive change rather than being simply reactive.

You will notice within the field of health care that for the many and varied roles, hierarchies and organisational tools and structures, capital letters are often used at the start of all words; examples of this might include Charge Nurse and Performance Improvement Plan. For greater ease of readability, however, capitals have not been used in this way in this book.

Note: the views within this book are mine, and do not represent the institutions in which I work. Staff reflections were sought from newly qualified nurses across the UK and their anonymity has been maintained.

Carol Forde-Johnston
September 2018

ACKNOWLEDGEMENTS

I would like to thank many people who have supported me over the years, but particularly my parents Clare and Jim Kirrane who instilled my work ethic and made me start a nursing course when I refused to stay on at school!

Thanks are also due to my husband James Forde-Johnston, sister Sharon Whitelaw and my mother- and father-in-law Kath and Alan Ridgway for their continual encouragement and support whilst working on this book.

Special thanks go to Anne Scott, Fiona Bond, Andrew Carter, Florian Stoermer, Dr Helen Walthall and Juliet Bostwick, who supported my development and allowed me the opportunity to work in a role developing others.

Finally, I need to thank my 8-year-old daughter Clodagh for putting up with my incessant typing over the last year and for just being you. I hope this book inspires you to reach for the stars and pursue a job you love, like Mummy.

The publishers would like to thank the following students and newly qualified nurses who contributed to the development of this book by reviewing draft contents and sample material. We have listed the universities they were attending during this process, although some will have graduated and registered as nurses since then.

Adam Cole – newly qualified nurse

Claire Douglas – Oxford Brookes University

Milena Krupinska – Oxford Brookes University

Niamh Lyons – Oxford Brookes University

Gerard Mawhinney – Oxford Brookes University

Louise Scott – University of Wolverhampton

ABBREVIATIONS

AD	advanced decisions	MDT	multidisciplinary team
AP	assistant practitioner	NA	nursing assistant
AVPU	alert, voice, pain, unresponsive	NEWS	National Early Warning Score
CCG	clinical commissioning group	NHS	National Health Service
CHPPD	care hours per patient day	NICE	National Institute for Health and Care Excellence
CN	charge nurse	NMC	Nursing and Midwifery Council
CPD	continuous practice development	NPOB	nurse per occupied bed
CQC	Care Quality Commission	NSI	nurse sensitive indicator
		OH	occupational health
CSW	clinical support worker	OT	occupational therapist
DNR	Do Not Resuscitate	PALS	Patient Advice and Liaison Service
DoLS	Deprivation of Liberty Safeguards	PIP	performance improvement plan
EWS	early warning scores	RCN	Royal College of Nursing
GCS	Glasgow Coma Scale		
HCA	health care assistant	RM	registered midwife
ICU	intensive care unit	RN	registered nurse
IMCA	independent mental capacity advocate	SNI	safe nursing indicator
KSF	Knowledge and Skills Framework	SW	support worker
		WTE	whole time equivalent
LP	lecturer practitioner		
LPA	lasting power of attorney		

CHAPTER 1

CHOOSING AND SECURING YOUR FIRST NURSING POST

❝ *I wish I had known that choosing the right first job, in an area with good clinical education and support, is so important. Fortunately I chose wisely! Even though I worked on a busy ward for my first year qualified, I had clinical educators to guide my learning and they made such a difference.* **❞**

3 years post-qualified children's nurse

❝ *I was not appointed to the post I really wanted and was devastated. I worked in a GP practice as a second year student and the staff all wanted me to come back once I had completed my training, so I just thought the job would be mine. Little did I know how popular the job would be, as two students from my cohort went for the same job and one of them got the post, as she interviewed much better than me. I was such an idiot for not prepping for that interview, but I picked myself up and decided to go for it again in a few years' time. I have another interview next week for a band 6 post and I have put hours into prepping for it this time.* **❞**

2 years qualified as ward staff nurse and 1 year as a
community staff nurse, his current post

As a lecturer practitioner, working in both a busy UK NHS trust and university, I offer advice every year to numerous student nurses and qualified nurses to help them choose the right job and secure the post in the area they want. I shortlist and interview for band 5 roles across my hospital division too, and the two questions I am most frequently asked by third year student nurses about to qualify are: *"How do I choose my first post?"* and *"Have you any interview tips to help me get the job I want?"* This chapter will try to answer these two key questions.

With preparation and by following the guidance and the interview tips in this chapter, you can achieve your goals and realise your aspirations!

1.1 HOW TO CHOOSE YOUR FIRST POST

The importance of your first post

The importance of choosing the *right* first nursing job, that offers support and opportunities to develop your future career, cannot be underestimated. I vividly remember my first post in the 1980s working on a busy neuro-surgical unit, where patients' beds were lined up, side by side, in a large open Nightingale ward that lacked privacy and had only a couple of side rooms. I remember rows of patients with full head shaves, as opposed to the partial head shave used prior to brain surgery today. I felt anxious when the charge nurse snapped: "*Staff nurse Kirrane, you won't get much done standing there!*" I remember feeling completely out of my depth and just wanting to turn around and go back to my cosy room in the nurses' home (all hospitals had very cheap nurses' accommodation back then). You were never called by your first name in the 1980s on UK hospital wards, and my students laugh when I tell them I had to stand to attention when my matron entered the vicinity. I remember odd smells, a strange mixture of smoke and antiseptic, from plumes of cigarette smoke enveloping the night nurse who was handing over to the morning staff while having the usual '*end of shift fag*' in the staff room. It all sounds alien today.

Although you are working in a different era, you will also have many successes and challenges during your first nursing post. You may make mistakes, small and large, as everyone does during their first year qualified. The importance of having a collaborative team to support you and good role models to nurture your development in your first post cannot be overstated.

I had an excellent senior staff nurse as a role model in my first post who taught me always to introduce myself to every patient, face to face, when I started my shift. I remember her explaining that if I focused on writing a care plan during the first hour of my shift, and not meeting patients, it would be very difficult to recognise a confused patient who might wander. I regularly used this simple advice given to me during my first year qualified caring for neurologically impaired patients, who often wandered around wards that had no security locks. On every shift that I have completed since, I always introduce myself to patients at the start of a shift and inform them when I am leaving.

Practical instruction that works, and which comes from a good nursing role model, never leaves you. When supporting newly qualified nurses caring for similar patients, I impart the same advice I was given 30 years ago. I also suggest that they ask relatives for permission to have a photo of the patient by their bedside, check local policies for caring for a confused patient who may wander, and discuss the ethics related to using an electronic 'wander guard' armband, along with the issues around consent and 'deprivation of liberty' that may be relevant to individual cases. Nursing care and your professional evidence base will always move forward and change with the times. You too will build on key advice given to you during your first year qualified as you progress through your nursing career.

The moral of the story and the point of my reminiscing:

> ❝ *Always take time and do your homework before choosing your first post. Check that the role will offer you a good standard of clinical education, a structured preceptorship programme and supportive role models to develop your skills. This will give you the best possible start to your future nursing career.* ❞

Nursing placements during your training

The way nurse training placements are set up, in busy hospital and community settings, with practice supervisors maintaining their normal caseloads, can make it difficult for newly qualified nurses to know exactly where to apply when they are near to qualifying. Some students experience a range of specialisms during their placements, such as surgery, medicine, outpatients, community, emergency care, rehabilitation, intensive care, theatres and end of life. They may know exactly which area they wish to pursue on qualification, whereas other students are unsure.

There is no need to worry just because a fellow student knows exactly which area they wish to start their career in and you don't. If you are uncertain about where to specialise, it may be helpful to structure your first post as a rotation post. Usually rotations are set up between two or three areas, and you spend 6 to 9 months in each area, although increasingly, health service employers are offering bespoke rotations, e.g. two areas over two years. A rotation does not suit all nurses as they can feel unsettled moving between areas. However, some new starters find rotations invaluable to help them decide which career pathway would be best for them in the long term.

Most UK health care employers realise that a newly qualified nurse is a valuable resource who is difficult to recruit and retain. You only have to scan the numerous band 5 nursing jobs advertised across the UK to see that it is *your market* and to *your advantage*. You should not demand in an interview that you must have a rotation, of course, but do not be afraid to ask for what you feel will develop your career to meet your needs, as well as the employer's.

Where to look for nursing jobs

When you decide to look for your first nursing post, there are a variety of places to scan for jobs. UK NHS employers advertise nursing jobs on national online recruitment sites aimed at health service personnel, such as *'NHS Jobs'* and *'NHS Scotland Recruitment'*. Jobs may also be found on other national online recruitment sites such as *'indeed.co.uk'*. However, it tends to be the private sector that uses these more generic recruitment sites. Health service employers also advertise in popular national nursing journals, local job centres and newspapers, or on noticeboards within their own institutions. In addition, the Royal College of Nursing (RCN) holds a number of national recruitment fairs across the UK for employers to market their jobs to applicants, and employers may also host their own local recruitment events.

What do you need to decide before you apply for your first post?

Answering the questions in *Box 1.1* may help you decide which post to apply for.

Further guidance is presented in *Table 1.1*, related to the questions in *Box 1.1*, to aid your decision-making.

The importance of an informal visit

The best way to establish whether a practice setting and the local team are going to support your individual needs is to arrange an informal visit. There is no standard practice for arranging an informal visit. You would usually start by contacting the nurse manager or sister/charge nurse (CN) by email or telephone, to secure an appropriate time. Remember that senior nurses need to prioritise the delivery of their services and you may

Box 1.1 Questions to help you choose where to apply for your first post

1. Do I know exactly where I want to work? (e.g. I enjoyed my placement so much as a student that I want to work in this area for the duration of my career)

2. Do I have to return home, or relocate, due to a partner or finances?

3. Do I have no idea where I want to work, but I know that I prefer a particular type of nursing? (e.g. surgery, medicine, rehab, intensive care or community health promotion)

4. Do I already know which role I want in the future and am I ambitious to secure that post as soon as possible? (e.g. specialist nurse, advanced nurse practitioner, nurse educator, research nurse, GP nurse, nurse consultant or alcohol advisor)

5. Do I have no idea where I want to work? (e.g. my placement experiences were too narrow or I cannot choose between a few interesting areas as they were all good)

not receive a response from a senior nurse for a few weeks if they are busy. It is advisable to include a deputy, team leader or practice educator in your email or telephone request, to increase your chance of an early response.

During an informal visit you can acquire a mass of information, and your observations and conversations with staff currently in post can greatly influence your decision on whether to apply or not. If you choose to apply, you can also use key information obtained during your visit to inform your answers at interview, e.g. the key priorities for nursing care required for patients in the related field or the nursing delivery system used.

I am surprised every year by the number of student nurses who apply for their first post and sign a contract with their employer without ever having actually visited the area beforehand. Work is a big part of your life, and to work 8- to 12-hour shifts in an area that you have not visited is taking a risk. During your first year qualified, you will need to consolidate everything that you have learnt during your nurse training, whilst also learning new extended skills. If you are happy because you find team members easy to work with, you have good role models and clear direction, then you will thrive during your first year. If the opposite is the case then

Table 1.1: Handy tips to guide your decision when applying for your first nursing post

Answers to the questions in *Box 1.1*	Guidance and tips
1. Yes, I know exactly where I want to work	If the area you are applying to is also a popular setting it will make the interview more competitive. If this is the perfect post for you, you need to prepare and plan for your interview rigorously (see interview guidance later in this chapter). Attend an informal visit in the area before your interview (see informal visit guidance later in this chapter).
2. Yes, I need to return home or relocate	Advice as above; however, you should check all suitable practice settings available to you, in and around your required location. I have occasional students every year who have struggled in the job that was nearest to where they live, only to find a more suitable post later a few miles away.
3. Yes, I know the area of nursing I prefer but I do not mind where I work	Although you are flexible, you should choose the area that will give you the most support and opportunities. Do your homework and find out as much as you can about all areas that offer suitable posts, e.g. arrange as many informal visits as you can across the range of available areas. Ask yourself key questions to help you decide, e.g. Can I work with the team in the area? Does the area offer me enough flexibility on the rota as I need one evening off per week? Are they offering me enough support and development during my first year? Were the new starters on the area positive about the support they had been given?
4. Yes, I know the role I am aiming for and am ambitious to start the role as soon as I can	Advice as above; however, your decision may also be based on the area that is most likely to offer you the quickest career pathway, i.e. the area that funds the most posts and relevant courses. Establish what qualifications are required for the post by speaking to nurses already established in the post, e.g. a *'nurse prescribing'* module for a specialist nurse or *'Masters'* for an advanced nurse practitioner or nursing sister / charge nurse. Establish which areas are most likely to offer you funding for a relevant course, as a university module will cost you hundreds of pounds if you decide to self-fund. Establish if there is a clear career pathway in the area to aid your development and progression, e.g. a band 5 leadership course to become a band 6.

Table 1.1: (Continued)

Answers to the questions in *Box 1.1*	Guidance and tips
5. Yes, I have no idea where I want to work or what nursing role I would like to do later in my career	Consider applying for a rotational post, e.g. 9 months in three different areas may be beneficial to help you decide which area you should pursue in your career.
	Alternatively, consider applying for a 1-year post that is the complete opposite to your student placements, to decide which type of nursing you really prefer, e.g. an oncology placement if you have had no previous placement experience of end of life / palliative / hospice care but you feel that it may be of interest to you.
	Arrange informal visits in a variety of different areas to observe the nurses with patients and get a 'feel' for a different area that may, or may not, suit your needs.
	Read around the different areas and specialities by reviewing employers' websites and ask for their new starter information and orientation packs – you can also watch online national videos from different specialist areas by staff, patient groups and charities.

you may struggle. My advice is to do your homework and not to take a risk in your first post.

An informal visit usually consists of an initial one-to-one meeting with a senior nurse or practice educator from the area to discuss what the post will offer you, the potential applicant. A one-to-one in the office is usually followed by a walk around the area, or a home visit / patient consultation if it is a community setting. I would be very wary of applying for any job, even now, if during an informal visit they would not allow me to have a walk around the work environment to talk to current staff. During your informal visit make sure that you talk to the manager, current experienced staff and new starters, about the area and support they offer (see *Table 1.2* for key questions to guide your informal visit). You can gain immense insight from current staff working in the role of band 5 during visits, which can inform your final choices later.

If you are applying for jobs that are miles away, it may not be feasible to conduct an informal visit. Alternatively, you can find out important information by having a telephone or Skype call with the nurse manager, or by accessing resources from the clinical educators via email. Always check which specific area you will be working in and ask for information about the actual post and the support that will be offered to you before

Table 1.2: Key questions to guide your informal visit

Questions during your informal visit	Rationale and helpful tips
1. What type of conditions do the patients have in the area and what special needs/requirements may they have?	You will gain insight into whether this area is appropriate and interesting enough for you to apply. You will gain increased insight to answer key interview questions, such as why you want a job here or what type of skills you have for the post. If there are a high number of patients with surgical wounds, for example, you may be asked about types of wounds. Do not be afraid to write notes during your informal visit as it shows your eagerness to learn.
2. Do you have practice educators, practice development nurses or clinical educators who support new starters? If yes, what support will they offer me when I start in my first month and during my first year? If not, do other staff offer this support and how is it delivered?	Areas that have dedicated nurse educators (areas will use different job titles) and a structured plan of support will be very helpful to your development during your first year, especially if you struggle during your initial transition from student to qualified nurse. Do not dismiss an area, however, that does not have a nurse educator role, as they may have excellent team leaders or deputy sisters/charge nurses who act as your preceptor during your first year qualified. Smaller nursing teams may not have the finances or need for such a role. Make sure that structured support is in place by asking staff how this support will be delivered during your first year. Be wary of applying for a first post if the senior nurse cannot answer how they are going to support you initially during your supernumerary period or during your first year.
3. Do you have a structured supernumerary period, orientation programme and preceptorship period? If so, what do they specifically entail?	Areas that aim to address and meet new starters' training and development needs will be able to explain what their area can offer you in relation to all three of these elements. Ask the senior nurse or clinical educator to email you their programmes of support if they do not have hard copies to show you on your visit. This will also be helpful if you want to compare offers across a number of potential posts from different areas.
4. Do you have a career pathway, study days or specialist education courses to help me progress in my band 5 role? Or into a future band 6 role in the next 2–3 years (if this is your goal when you qualify)?	You may not want to move to a band 6 post, which is fine; however, you should have access to future study days and courses to support your learning and future development as a band 5 over the next 2–3 years in post. If you are ambitious and are striving for a future band 6 post, do not be afraid to ask whether the area will support your ambitions and determine how the area will actively do this.

Table 1.2: (Continued)

Questions during your informal visit	Rationale and helpful tips
5. **Relevant questions linked to your specific learning or social needs**	Does the area provide flexibility to meet your specific learning needs and/or social life/lifestyle?
	Write your own questions to meet your needs, e.g. can the rota accommodate your once-weekly hobby? Can I continue to pick my children up from school? How many weekends will I have to work?

NOTE: *The above questions can also be used during a booked Skype/telephone interview.* Questions 2–5 *may be asked during your actual interview; however, you should know the answer to* Question 1 *before you apply for the post.*

you arrive for interview. You should be offered an extensive orientation as a new starter nurse and you can request a Skype call and ask for copies of new starter orientation packs and study days to be sent to you via email. If they are not forthcoming following repeated requests, then consider applying elsewhere.

Most NHS employers have a 6-month probationary period for all bands of staff to assess whether they are up to the job once appointed. Line managing a new starter out of a job is a worst case scenario and rarely happens, but it can occur. To prevent the risk of future disciplinary disputes, try to make sure that you are going to work in an area that is going to develop your confidence with structured support.

In summary, whether you attend an informal visit, or have contact via telephone or Skype, I would always advise that you avoid any area that does not offer you a new starter orientation or structured plan of support when you commence your first nursing post, as they do not deserve to have you without this in place!

1.2 YOUR APPLICATION AND PERSONAL STATEMENT

Here are a few tips for writing your application and personal statement:

- Ensure that you complete your application in time for the deadline as you will not be shortlisted after this date. Most applications are centralised through a Human Resources (HR) department, which makes it impossible to upload an application once the deadline has expired.

- Make sure that your application is neat and concise, and does not contain spelling or grammatical errors. Ask friends, family, university academic advisors and peers to proofread your application prior to submission.

- Do not falsify any data on your application as HR staff are trained to check the details and rigorous referencing checks will pick up inconsistencies.

- Take time to write a personal statement that is personal to you and shows your strengths.

- Your personal statement should make reference to the following three areas:
  - the importance of compassionate patient care and how you strive to deliver individualised, holistic, patient-focused care
  - the importance of maintaining professional standards and how you aim to achieve this
  - how well you work in a team and what you can offer your future employer.

Although managers will have individual areas they are interested in, these are the three key areas that most nurse managers will be looking for in a band 5 application.

- Always use language that you understand and are comfortable with, and do not just copy material that you read online or in books that you 'think' should be in a personal statement.

1.3 PREPARING FOR BAND 5 INTERVIEWS

There are some key areas that will be covered by interviewers during band 5 interviews; even if interviewers word their questions differently they will be probing for some key information from the candidates through their questioning. *Table 1.3* provides details as to what interviewers are usually looking for, and some example band 5 questions are presented to help you prepare for your interview.

You should also prepare for any potential spontaneous questions in your band 5 interview. Usually these are linked to current health care topics from media and nursing journals, so you should review current nursing journals and listen to the news channels for a period leading up to your interview for potential 'hot' topics. Current areas would include development of the new band 4 nursing associate role and changes to professional standards, e.g. 2018 NMC standards: *Future Nurse: standards of proficiency for registered nurses* (NMC, 2018a) and standards for education and training, presented in three parts (NMC, 2018b; NMC, 2018c; NMC, 2018d).

Often I interview band 5s as the third interviewer, and when most key questions (*Table 1.3*) have been asked in some form by the first two interviewers, I will ask questions linked to something that the candidate mentioned earlier in the interview or wrote in their personal statement. If you say or write that you always provide *'evidence-based practice'* or adhere to *'clinical governance systems'*, then you should be able to answer questions on these terms in your interview, i.e. what they mean and how you achieve this. Every year I interview nurses who have no idea what terms such as these actually mean, when they are claiming within their personal statements that they are embedded in their practice. Make sure that you understand everything that you write on your application.

When responding to questions, keep to what you know best and be yourself. A caring person who is a team player will come across well in an interview even if they stumble over words and cannot quite articulate everything clearly. It is always evident if an interviewee is just using health care buzzwords and does not really understand the words they are using.

It is important that you review your placement feedback from past practice supervisors and that you prepare key examples from practice linked to patients, or relevant situations that you have had to deal with where you can show off any key skills required for the band 5 post. Just one good example linked to compassionate care, team working, maintaining quality and/or professional standards, or dealing with a challenging situation will see you through any band 5 interview.

Many employers use values-based interviewing, where they will ask all candidates the same few non-specific open questions, e.g. *"Can you define compassionate care for us?"* The interviewer will expect a relevant example from your practice that shows you understand the question. If you are called to a *'values-based'* band 5 interview always ensure that you have good examples that detail exactly what you did in a given scenario related to the question. Usually, values-based questions will relate to one of the areas given in *Table 1.3*. It is advisable to choose one good example from practice during your training that demonstrates your skills related to each area in *Table 1.3*. If you are not used to this style of interviewing and open questioning, preparing a good example

Table 1.3: Example band 5 interview questions

What the interviewer is looking for	Example band 5 questions
The role/service you are applying for	
Whether you are interested in the role/area/service and that you know enough about the job that you have applied for Whether you are genuinely interested and keen, as you are more likely to say yes if offered the post	1. What interested you in the post/role? 2. Why do you want a role within our unit/service? 3. Why do you want to work in this area/service as opposed to anywhere else? 4. From the job description, what do you feel are the main aspects of the role? 5. What key skills are needed within the role? 6. What skills do you have to offer for the role? 7. What is your understanding of the trust values/service mission statement and why are they important? 8. *Question relating to specific care in the area:* What do you know about the waiting list targets in our A&E area? *(NOTE: use your informal visit or Skype/phone call to find out any related details specific to the area/post)*
Compassionate, individualised, holistic, patient-focused care	
Whether you have an ability to provide compassionate, individualised, holistic and patient-focused care Whether you come across as a kind, empathetic person who will meet the needs of the patients in their service who you will be caring for Whether you make judgements and label patients or their families, which means you would not be suitable for their service	1. Give us an example of when you last provided compassionate care to one of the patients you cared for *(NOTE: the interviewer may use any one of the terms compassionate, individualised, holistic and patient-focused within any of the questions in this section. If you choose a good example or two from your past practice they would answer any of these framed questions)* 2. How would you define compassionate *(or holistic/patient-centred)* care?

Whether you respect equality and diversity laws and do not discriminate against a person's sex, gender, disability, sexual orientation, religion, belief, race or age	3. How do you deliver compassionate care? 4. What hinders compassionate care and how would you overcome barriers to compassionate care?

Good communicator and a team player

Whether you are a good communicator who would communicate well with patients and team members within their service Whether you have the qualities to fit in with the service / team you will be working with (NOTE: this works both ways as I have been to interviews where I refused the job offered due to what was said in the interview about the way a team worked, which I knew would not fit with my style of working)	1. What is your understanding of good communication skills? 2. Give us an example of communication methods you might use when caring for a patient who had difficulty communicating their needs 3. What is your understanding of team work and being a team player? 4. What specific skills do you have to offer our service / team / the role? 5. Talk me through a time when you had to deal with a problem in a team or you witnessed challenges within a team – talk through how these challenges were overcome

Coping with the stresses of the job

Whether you can identify when you are becoming stressed and know how to ask for help when you are unsure of care or need extra support Whether you are a safe nurse, i.e. you do not deliver care if you are ever unsure, you know how to delegate appropriately to nursing assistants and to escalate concerns appropriately Whether you know how to access support and who to escalate concerns to when needed Whether you know how to prevent stress and deal with stress related to the role Whether you will cope with a band 5 role within their service / area	1. What tools do you use to help you prioritise your workload? 2. How do you know when to escalate concerns? 3. What tools do you use to escalate patient concerns? 4. What would you do if one of your patients deteriorated? (NOTE: often an example will be given linked to a relevant scenario from the area that may need escalating) 5. Can you give us an example of a time when you managed a difficult situation and tell us what the outcome was? 6. What are your strengths and weaknesses? 7. What would be the most worrying part of being a band 5 if you were offered the post?

(continued)

Table 1.3: (*Continued*)

What the interviewer is looking for	Example band 5 questions
	8. What aspects of a trained nurse role do you feel will make you most stressed when you qualify?
	9. How do you know when you are becoming stressed? How do you manage stress? How do you prevent yourself from becoming stressed?
	10. How do you plan to cope with your first patient caseload?
	11. How do you plan to delegate to nursing assistants when you start a band 5 role?
	12. Explain how you delegate as a student and link to a specific clinical example
Professional standards, quality care and safety	
Whether you can maintain high professional standards underpinned by an appropriate evidence base	1. How do you keep up to date?
Whether you have knowledge of correct practice, risk assessments and national policies	2. What does evidence-based practice mean to you?
Whether you would adhere to national safeguarding directives and legislation	3. What does quality care mean to you?
Whether you are a liability to their service, e.g. you have poor standards that could lead to poor care within their service and potential future complaints and litigation	4. Give us an example from practice where you have delivered quality care / evidence-based practice
	5. Some interviewers will test you by giving you a scenario to check whether you would be a safe practitioner, e.g. if a patient was in severe pain and begged you to give them analgesics that were not prescribed, would you give them this medication without a medical prescription? (*NOTE: the answer is NO; you would escalate this situation for urgent medical review to ensure the patient was not left in pain, unless the registered nurse is a qualified 'nurse prescriber' who is allowed to prescribe the medication prior to administration* (NMC, 2018a).)

beforehand can make you feel less uncomfortable and help you avoid going off at a tangent and not answering a values-based question specifically enough.

As well as preparing for key questions, here are a few more tips for your band 5 interview:

Always arrive in plenty of time

- I advise arriving an hour before the start of any interview to ensure you arrive in the right place. You will then have time to go to the toilet, or have a coffee, and will not be rushed and panicked at the start of your interview. You will be nervous enough without adding any further pressures on yourself.

- If you have had to deal with an unforeseeable delay or sickness, ensure that you contact the interviewers by phone and email as soon as possible. If you let them know you will be late or not able to attend they may be able to rejig their schedules and offer you a later interview that day. They are also much more likely to offer another interview date if you cancel prior to the interview, rather than just not turning up for interview and requesting an interview days later.

Present yourself well and try to calm any nerves through good preparation

- Dress cleanly and smartly and try to smile and be approachable, even if you are nervous.

- If you are really nervous just be honest and let the interviewers know. They should not be trying to trip you up, as you are new to the profession and probably will not have had many interviews. Remember everyone is nervous when they are interviewed.

- Most interviewers will try to put you at ease and attempt to get the best answers out of you at interview.

- Rarely, interviewers will try to show off, or are stressed in their role or new to interviewing, and may be rather nervous or wound up. This may lead them to ask a candidate a complicated question in two or three parts. If this happens in your interview, never be afraid to ask the interviewer to clarify what they are asking you, to ensure you understand the question.

The more prepared you feel in your interview, the less nervous you will be. You can ask friends, peers and past practice supervisors to give you a mock interview and honest feedback on your answers. Use *Table 1.3* for guidance on potential interview questions.

The rating of your interviews according to your answers

All interviewers should record the candidate's answers, to ensure parity and equity across the interviews that are taking place. Usually employers and institutions have a standard interview record form to complete for each candidate. Many of these forms use rating scales and scores to provide feedback on each answer given by each candidate, and the sum of these will lead to a total score at the end of the interview. A '0' score would be given where the candidate gave an incorrect answer or a poor answer with no tangible evidence, or a hypothetical answer with no substance. In contrast, a very well answered question may receive a score of '3' indicating that the answer exceeded all criteria being measured or the question was positively answered with excellent patient examples, or no concerns were noted.

If you are unsuccessful at interview, make sure you request interview feedback from the lead interviewer. Their feedback will help inform your future interview preparation and identify the key questions you need to work on.

REFERENCES

Nursing and Midwifery Council (2018a) *Future Nurse: standards of proficiency for registered nurses.* Available at: www.nmc.org.uk/globalassets/sitedocuments/education-standards/future-nurse-proficiencies.pdf (last accessed 10 June 2018)

Nursing and Midwifery Council (2018b) *Realising Professionalism: standards for education and training Part 1: Standards framework for nursing and midwifery education.* Available at: www.nmc.org.uk/globalassets/sitedocuments/education-standards/education-framework.pdf (last accessed 10 June 2018)

Nursing and Midwifery Council (2018c) *Realising Professionalism: standards for education and training Part 2: Standards for student supervision and assessment.* Available at: www.nmc.org.uk/globalassets/sitedocuments/education-standards/student-supervision-assessment.pdf (last accessed 10 June 2018)

Nursing and Midwifery Council (2018d) *Realising Professionalism: standards for education and training Part 3: Standards for pre-registration nursing programmes.* Available at: www.nmc.org. uk/globalassets/sitedocuments/education-standards/programme-standards-nursing.pdf (last accessed 10 June 2018)

WHAT TO DO NEXT

1. Put time and effort into choosing the right first post to meet your development needs when you qualify. Ensure that you choose an area/post that has a good standard of clinical education, a structured orientation and preceptorship programme, and supportive role models, to develop your clinical skills.

2. Make sure you find out whether the post/area is right for you by attending an informal visit. If this is not possible organise a Skype/phone meeting with the nurse manager and nurse educator. Do not apply for an area if this support is not forthcoming or evident.

3. Ensure that you ask for copies of orientation packs and new starter study days/programmes of support before you apply for your band 5 post.

4. Establish what education courses and career pathways are supported within the areas/role you are thinking of applying for, to aid your decision-making.

5. Don't be afraid to ask for rotations, to enable you to decide which area would be best for you to develop your long-term career, if you are unsure on qualification.

6. Put time and effort into preparing for your band 5 interview and always have specific examples that you can recall at interview to show off your key transferable skills, e.g. linked to communication, compassion, team working, quality, standards, dealing with challenges in the workplace and resilience.

7. Research 'hot topics' within the profession and have a clear understanding of current professional standards prior to interview.

CHAPTER 2

STRUCTURING YOUR LEARNING DURING YOUR FIRST THREE MONTHS QUALIFIED

❝ *I wish I had known that I needed to be more assertive when I started my ward orientation and not be afraid to ask questions. I was given an orientation pack but I did not know what to prioritise. I should have asked for specific advice on which study days were essential and which could have been left until my second year. I focused too much on trying to learn everything, instead of focusing on essential statutory training and e-learning in those first two weeks.* ❞

2 years post-qualified ward nurse

❝ *Constructive feedback is essential during your first few months as this is where you develop your competence and key skills, and it helps set the foundation for your future development. It is very important to establish who will give you clinically sound and honest advice within your team. I was allocated a fantastic band 6 deputy charge nurse to look after me that made such a difference.* ❞

1 year post-qualified mental health nurse

When making the transition from third year student to newly qualified nurse you may feel a mix of emotions. I remember my parents being incredibly proud that their rebellious daughter, who refused to do her A levels, was now a State Registered Nurse moving to Cambridge. I felt excited at the prospect of moving away from my childhood home in Coventry to a *'posher place full of bikes and academics'*, but also scared of having to *'go it alone in the real world'*. In the 1980s we were paid a wage during our nurse training and as a first year I received £128 in my first month's pay packet. I was always counted in the staffing numbers during my placements, as we were classed as paid workers from the local *'School of Nursing'*. During my final year, I had to be signed off as competent when taking charge of a 28-bedded ward, which gave me a taster of what to expect when qualified.

Paying student nurses as part of the NHS workforce contrasts with the supernumerary status student nurses have today. You will always have worked under direct supervision and never been solely accountable for the care of your patients. Many newly qualified nurses contact me to discuss their immense sense of achievement at having gained a professional qualification, whilst voicing concerns about their fear of the unknown. You are, however, more highly educated than nurses from the past, being trained to think critically and problem-solve, which enables you to make highly complex decisions to match current health care challenges.

In my experience, newly qualified nurses' concerns usually relate to two key questions: *"What do I need to learn first, as there is so much to learn?"* and *"How do I structure my learning in the first few months?"* This chapter attempts to answer these important questions, offering guidance as to what you can expect, what to focus on during your orientation period, and how to structure your learning.

2.1 WHAT TO EXPECT WHEN YOU START

Initial nerves and anxieties

You are probably feeling nervous about what lies ahead and these are normal anxieties that many new nurses experience. Try not to place pressure on yourself to perform to the highest standards or worry about your lack of knowledge. You have worked extremely hard for three years and should commend yourself for balancing your degree course work with professional competencies, which is not an easy feat. If you have already been awarded a nursing degree, or are near to qualifying, then you *must* have the potential skills to become a competent qualified nurse and no one expects you to know it all!

Knowing what to expect during your first few months qualified, and approaching learning in a methodical way, will help decrease your anxieties. Identifying your specific learning needs, formulating individual objectives or goals, questioning and reflecting on your own practice, and working on feedback from your preceptor should become an inherent part of your first year qualified. You may seek additional support through a variety of ways if you struggle at any time through your career. *Chapter 9* details how to deal with a lack of progression, and identifies strategies to prevent and manage stress as you take on more responsibilities.

Your induction and essential training

Before you start in practice, your employer should always offer you an induction. Your induction should include, as a minimum, *statutory training that is required for you to practise, as defined by current national health and safety regulations.* Currently, the minimum statutory training required for trained nurses includes the following areas:

- Fire safety
- Equality and diversity
- Health and safety awareness
- Information governance
- Manual handling.

Your manager will ask you to attend statutory training study days, which may be delivered in a classroom, lecture theatre or simulation laboratory. You may be asked to complete workbooks, quizzes or online e-learning packages, to ensure that you comply and pass the required level when assessed. It is important that you *complete all statutory training* prior to working in the practice setting, as you may not be fully covered by insurers to practise without adequate training.

In contrast to statutory training, *mandatory training is compulsory and determined by your employer.* Mandatory training is based on your nursing responsibilities and job description, as opposed to health and safety regulations. Often health care providers use the terms '*compulsory*' or '*essential*' training interchangeably to cover both statutory and mandatory training, which they expect you to complete within a certain time frame. Training aims to reduce the risk of mistakes and poor practice within an organisation by complying with national and government guidelines.

Always check with your line manager which mandatory training is required as part of your specific role. Mandatory training may include areas such as:

- adult/children hospital life support
- blood glucose monitoring
- blood safety and safe blood transfusion

- child protection and safeguarding children
- clinical record-keeping
- complaints handling
- conflict resolution
- consent and mental capacity
- electronic patient records
- safe administration of insulin
- infection prevention and control
- safeguarding adults
- medical devices
- venous thromboembolism.

Your first training priority will be to identify what statutory and mandatory training you need to complete and when it must be completed. If your employer uses an e-learning system you will automatically receive email alerts if you have not completed your training on time. If you are unsure which training is mandatory or statutory, you should contact your manager or practice educator who should advise you.

To help prioritise your statutory and mandatory training when you qualify, you may use a simple checklist (see example checklist in *Table 2.1*).

Supernumerary time and your orientation

There are no nationally recognised clinical training outcomes for newly qualified nurses. You should, however, always have a *specified period of induction* and an *orientation to your practice setting*, which should include *supernumerary time*. Supernumerary time, where your presence at work is not counted in the rota numbers, allows you time to complete essential training and to familiarise yourself with the clinical setting.

In my experience, I have never known a clinical setting not to give their newly qualified nurses a set number of supernumerary days as part of their orientation to acclimatise to their new role. There is, however, a great variety in the amount of supernumerary time awarded across clinical settings, which can range from a few days to several weeks, or months in some intensive care areas. Your employer is not obliged to give you supernumerary time to complete your statutory and mandatory training. Many managers do, however, allocate a number of induction study days to

Table 2.1: *Example paperwork to guide your statutory and mandatory training*

Type of training	Mandatory (M) or statutory (S)	How often	Expiry date	E-learning or workbook	Assessment or online quiz	Classroom or skills session	Date all completed	Notes
Fire safety	S	Yearly	31.03.19	✓ 1.02.18	✓ 31.03.18	✓ 31.03.18	1.04.18	
Manual handling theory	S	3-yearly	31.03.21	✓ 1.02.18	✓ 31.03.18		1.04.18	
Manual handling practical	S	3-yearly	31.03.21	n/a	n/a	Await practical session		Only managed half the session due to an emergency on the ward, second half booked next week 1st April
Information governance	S	Yearly	31.03.19	✓ 1.02.18	✓ 31.03.18		1.04.18	
Equality and diversity	S	3-yearly	31.03.21	✓ 1.02.18	✓ 31.03.18		1.04.18	
Health and safety	S	3-yearly	31.03.21	✓ 1.02.18	✓ 31.03.18		1.04.18	
Safeguarding/protection of vulnerable adults	M	3-yearly	31.03.21	✓ 1.02.18	✓ 31.03.18		1.04.18	
Safeguarding children level 1	M	3-yearly	31.03.21	✓ 1.02.18	✓ 31.03.18		1.04.18	
Infection control	M	2-yearly	31.03.20	✓ 1.02.18	✓ 31.03.18		1.04.18	

NOTE: *The information in this table is to be used ONLY as an example and you may require additional training. Always check up-to-date training requirements with your line manager.*

enable their staff to complete essential training and familiarise themselves with the role. It is always wise to find out how much supernumerary time will be offered to you before you decide on your first post.

Similarly, there is a lack of standardisation relating to the structure and content of orientation programmes for newly qualified nurses across the UK. They may range from a few pages of local information to an in-depth competency-based orientation as part of a year-long preceptorship programme. It is important that you determine what is expected of you during your orientation period, along with time frames for completion.

An example of a comprehensive orientation checklist, identifying key information required before you start your first post, is presented in *Table 2.2*. This checklist may guide your orientation, although it is not exhaustive, and you may wish to personalise it to meet your individual needs.

2.2 HOW TO STRUCTURE YOUR LEARNING IN YOUR FIRST FEW MONTHS QUALIFIED

Preceptorship

The Department of Health (DH, 2010) and the NMC (2008) advise that newly qualified nurses should have a period of structured preceptorship, to help their transition from student to qualified nurse or midwife. The aim of preceptorship is to support the newly qualified nurse to consolidate their skills gained as a student, to enable them to become confident and competent future practitioners. During the preceptorship period, the newly qualified nurse (the preceptee) will be supported by one trained nurse (their preceptor) within their clinical setting. In reality, it is not always feasible for a newly qualified nurse to be able to work every shift with their preceptor, over the full preceptorship period. If preceptors are not available, shift 'buddies' may be allocated, to provide assurance that there is a trained nurse available for support.

You will require regular support and guidance from an experienced nurse, who should act as a positive role model, to enable you to develop your professional skills. During your supernumerary time, you should familiarise yourself with key routines in your clinical setting, and observe experienced nurses at work, until you are confident enough to take your own caseload. Prior to taking a caseload, you should be allocated a 'buddy' on every shift who acts as a support during your supernumerary time. You

Table 2.2: Orientation checklist

Key areas	Specific information	Completed
Statutory and mandatory training	List of statutory and mandatory training (required first few weeks to 3 months post-qualification)	
	Training booking system and how to navigate	
	Online learning system to access workbooks / e-learning	
Roles and responsibilities	List of roles within the nursing team (trained and untrained) and responsibilities (*Chapter 3*)	
	List of roles within the allied health professions and responsibilities	
	Organisational structures within the institution, trust or community setting	
	System for patient allocation and delegation of caseloads (*Chapters 3* and *4*)	
Policies	Location of national and local policies / standards	
	Policy to book rota requests, study days, annual / compassionate leave	
Documentation	Documentation required for patient pathways (admission to discharge)	
	Observation charts	
	Pre-op checklists	
	Consent forms	
	Acuity and dependency tools (*Chapter 4*)	
	Paperwork less frequently used, e.g. self-discharge, Deprivation of Liberty, registering death, storing valuables, assessing mental capacity and Do Not Resuscitate (DNR) forms	
	Systems to document care, e.g. electronic patient records	
	Standardised care plans (*Chapter 7*)	
Risk assessments	National and local risk assessment documentation (*Chapter 6*)	
Human resources (HR)	HR team and their location	
	Uniform policy	
	Key employer policies, e.g. performance and conduct, bullying and harassment	
Orientating to the service	Layout of the setting (or region if community nurse)	
	Position of setting relative to other health care providers	

(continued)

Table 2.2: (Continued)

Key areas	Specific information	Completed
	Type of handovers, e.g. patient bedside handover, written, taped recorded, MDT (multidisciplinary team)	
	Location of handover, emergency equipment and fire exits	
	Security in the clinical/community setting, e.g. security codes, safety bleeps/personal alarm	
	Storage of patient notes	
	Type of nursing organisational system used, e.g. team nursing (*Chapter 3*)	
	Key telephone numbers/contacts, e.g. specialist nurses	
	Referral system to doctors and allied health professionals	
	Patient call bell system	
	Shift patterns and breaks	
	System for reporting sickness	
Bleeping and escalation	National Early Warning scoring system and escalation policy (*Chapter 8*)	
	Escalation system relating to poor care	
Incident reporting	System to report incidents and escalate concerns (*Chapter 8*)	
	Procedure for preventing and reporting injury, e.g. a needlestick injury	
Medication and pharmacy	Common medications used in the setting, their actions/side-effects	
	Location of pharmacy/pharmacist	
	System to contact pharmacist (normal hours/out of hours)	
	Controlled drug and medication storage	
	Medication ordering and prescribing	
	Drug administration policy and procedure for reporting drug error	
	Patient self-administration medication policy (if appropriate)	
Equipment training	List of equipment used and where stored/cleaned/maintained	
	How to use equipment and training required (check whether additional training required to use equipment or you need observation/sign-off as competent)	
Patient information	Types of patients and common conditions	
	Usual patient pathways (referral to discharge)	
	Patient information packs (leaflets and standardised care plans)	

Table 2.2: (Continued)

Key areas	Specific information	Completed
Competencies and training	Induction and orientation programme	
	Preceptorship period and how delivered	
	Person signing you off as competent (line manager and/or preceptor)	
	System for practice review over 12 months	
	Band 5 skills required over first year and training, e.g. role-specific competencies/objectives	
	Systems of support in practice, e.g. observational feedback/action learning/group forums	
	Appraisal system	

NOTE: *The information in this table is to be used ONLY as an example and you may require changes/additions/deletions, according to service needs. Always check up-to-date training requirements with your line manager.*

will be expected to observe experienced nurses to increase your knowledge and 'learn whilst on the job'.

There is no mandatory requirement for employers to deliver preceptorship, as it is only *'strongly recommended'* by the Nursing and Midwifery Council (NMC, 2008). No professional or government body regularly monitors the implementation of preceptorship across the UK, leading to widespread differences in its implementation. The preceptorship period may last anywhere from 3 to 12 months post-qualification, and implementation has also been found to be variable as a result of staff shortages and service demands.

There are a number of key terms relating to the implementation of preceptorship:

Preceptorship

- A structured period of 'transition' for a newly registered practitioner where they are supported by a *'preceptor'*, to develop their confidence and skills in practice, as part of their lifelong learning. Note: the term *'preceptorship'* is not just related to nurses, as all allied health professionals are advised to have a period of preceptorship post-qualification.

- Preceptorship involves a *'preceptor'* supporting a *'preceptee'* in their clinical setting by providing an opportunity to reflect on practice, receive constructive feedback and have access to relevant post-registration learning.
- Preceptorship should be guided by role-specific competencies and an individualised development programme.

Preceptorship period

- The initial period after registration, and during a *preceptee's* first appointment as a qualified nurse, is referred to as the *'preceptorship period'*.
- There is no standard time frame for the preceptorship period, which can range from a few months to a year. The NMC (2008) and DH (2010) advise that the preceptorship period should last up to one year.

Preceptee

- A *preceptee* is a newly qualified nurse, midwife or allied health professional who is allocated a *'preceptor'* to support their development in a practice setting. From the first day of their appointment a *preceptee* should be allocated a named *preceptor*.

Preceptor

- A *preceptor* is a named member of qualified staff who is allocated to support a *preceptee's* development during their preceptorship period, usually up to a year.
- The *preceptor* must be based in the clinical setting, have been qualified at least a year and have experience of supervising others.
- The *preceptor* does not have to have a teaching/mentoring qualification, but must have good knowledge of the area.
- The *preceptor* is responsible for providing a newly qualified nurse with structured support in clinical practice during their preceptorship period.

It remains the responsibility of local health providers to decide the length and level of preceptorship to be delivered. It is important to establish whether preceptorship is offered within your practice setting and how it will be implemented during your first year qualified, e.g. who will be your preceptor and whether you have role-specific competencies that your preceptor will need to sign off.

A form to guide feedback from your preceptor, or shift buddy, is presented in *Box 2.1*. If you have a busy shift or caseload, it may be helpful for you to fill in key details prior to starting, such as your past experience and goals for the shift.

Box 2.1 **Example feedback form for newly qualified nurse / midwife**

Preceptorship practice feedback form for newly qualified nurse / midwife

Name of preceptee:

Name of preceptor / shift practice supervisor:

Date and time of shift:

Is the preceptee supernumerary on shift: YES / NO (please circle)

Ward area / community setting / clinical setting:

Overall aim(s) for feedback on this shift	*(e.g. to develop the nurse's time management skills when caring for a caseload or to improve skills of medicines management…)*
Detail your previous experience and what feedback will help you during this shift	*(State how many weeks / months you have been qualified and the specific feedback that would help your development. Both the preceptor and preceptee need to be clear what the aim of feedback is.)*

Following your shift, please reflect on what you did well and what needs to be improved.

Also detail what additional support will help improve your practice:

Preceptor / shift practice supervisor: please give feedback on the nurse's performance during the shift, detailing what the nurse did well and what their strengths were:

Please summarise and bullet-point key areas for the nurse to work on in the future using joint goal planning:

Please detail any additional support and training that you have suggested that may develop the nurse in the future:

Signature of preceptee: Date:

Signature of preceptor /   Date:
shift buddy:

Role-specific competencies

You are responsible and accountable for maintaining your professional competence when qualified, and your employer will need to be assured that you are competent to practise. You will have completed numerous competencies throughout your training as mentors or practice supervisors/practice assessors assessed your 'knowledge', 'skills' and 'values', the three core elements of any competency-based framework. The NMC (2008) advocates that all newly qualified nurses should also complete role-specific competencies post-qualification, during their preceptorship period, to develop their skills as part of their lifelong learning. New NMC (2018) *'proficiencies'* grouped under *'7 platforms'* and *'procedural competencies'* specify the knowledge and skills that newly qualified nurses must achieve to qualify before caring for *'people of all ages and across all care settings'*. Some clinical settings do not provide band 5 role-specific competencies, as they can be complicated and time-consuming to write. If your clinical setting does not provide specific competencies, you can write your own individual learning aims, objectives or 'SMART' goals, as part of your professional development plan. Your future development and revalidation at 1 year post-qualification are discussed in further detail in *Chapter 9*.

Many employers use e-learning training systems that involve the completion of online workbooks and quizzes to assure staff compliance with essential training. They are assured that the nurse has been given the correct theory to underpin their evidence base and has passed a quiz to assess their knowledge to practise safely. E-learning packages often state that they *'will enable you to demonstrate competence'*; however, in my view competence is not just about passing a quiz; it is also about your practical application of this theory. Competence is best assessed in your practice setting by an experienced nurse observing and reviewing your developing skills over your first year qualified. Role-specific competencies, SMART goals or learning objectives may help to structure your preceptor's assessment and feedback after you have been observed in practice.

In summary, it is important to establish which assessment and review methods your clinical setting will use to support your development during your first few months qualified. You should proactively develop your own SMART goals or learning objectives, if there are none in place when you start, and request regular feedback from your preceptor as part of your future professional development plan.

Aims, learning objectives and SMART goals

During your first few months qualified, it is helpful to structure your overall learning using development aims, learning objectives or SMART goals, especially if there are no role-specific competencies provided. Firstly, check whether your clinical setting provides orientation packs with core objectives and goals already written for you, as some do.

When you qualify you can easily become overwhelmed by the amount to learn and the different terms used to describe your learning and development. If you use a methodical approach, such as writing achievable learning objectives for 3-monthly reviews, you can feel more confident that you are positively developing your clinical knowledge and practice. In my experience, many newly qualified nurses struggle with writing their own SMART goals or learning objectives. Some questions that newly qualified nurses regularly ask me are shown below, together with key terms and guidance to help you if you have to write your own goals in the future.

What is a developmental aim and how does it differ from a learning objective?

There is usually one overall teaching, training or development aim (you can think of it as one strategy), whereas there will be a number of objectives (things to do) to complete the aim. The aim is usually an overall statement of intent that relates to specific objectives or goals set.

An example aim and learning objectives are presented in *Box 2.2*, relating to the delivery of a one-hour teaching session. It is up to the teacher to decide which objectives should be focused on here and there could potentially be different objectives that could link to the aim in *Box 2.2*. The teacher is mindful of what can be realistically achieved in one hour, what is important relating to students' current level of knowledge, and how student learning can be assessed. Similarly, your own learning objectives for the first month, and up to 3 months qualified, should be:

Box 2.2 Example teaching aim and objectives

AIM: the student will be able to increase their knowledge and understanding of the anatomy and physiology of the brain.

OBJECTIVES: the student will be able to:

- state the four lobes of the brain and describe their function
- identify the arteries of the circle of Willis and describe how they supply the structures and lobes of the brain
- define the different types of nerves in the brain and their functions
- explain the role of neurotransmitters and how electrical conduction takes place within the brain.

- focused on your individual learning needs and the requirements and responsibilities in your new role
- realistically timetabled to enable you to achieve the objectives by completion dates
- measurable, for you to know when they have been achieved.

What are learning objectives and how do I write them?

Learning objectives (sometimes called learning outcomes) are statements that describe what you need to be able to do, as a result of your learning. The aims will usually include general words such as 'know', 'understand', 'use' or 'show', whereas your objectives will use 'active verbs' to demonstrate their achievement, such as 'list', 'state', 'explain', 'discuss' or 'describe'.

Nursing is not just a theoretical profession as it involves practical skills and attitudes. *Box 2.3* contains some 'active verbs' associated with knowledge, skills and attitudes that may be used within your future learning objectives.

Box 2.3 Example of verbs to use in learning objectives

Overall aim	Example verbs for your learning objectives
KNOWLEDGE: to be able to demonstrate increased knowledge and understanding of ...	identify, define, state, interpret, list, label, classify, outline, record, evaluate, compare, recognise, calculate, label
SKILL: to be able to competently ...	use, locate, employ, maintain, measure, observe, chart, establish, interact, modify
ATTITUDES: to be able to demonstrate attitudes or values that reflect ...	value, support, consider, evaluate, challenge, characterise

Before you write your own aims and learning objectives during your first few months qualified, you need to know what should be prioritised. Within your first few weeks, for example, you may be required to competently use all manual handling aids, or a child's monitor, or safely complete depression risk assessments, before you take a caseload of patients. Always write your aims and objectives for your first few months qualified with the guidance of your preceptor, to ensure you identify the correct priorities relating to your roles and key responsibilities. An example nursing aim and objectives for your first few weeks qualified are presented in *Box 2.4*. Active verbs within the learning objectives have been highlighted in bold and your understanding and skill will be measured on the behaviours and tasks related to these active verbs.

Box 2.4 Example nursing aim and objective

Aim	Objectives (active verbs have been highlighted in **bold**)
To understand the roles and responsibilities of health care professionals in my clinical setting and how they relate to the service	• **Review** my job description and **identify** my key role and responsibilities as a newly qualified nurse • **List** all health care professional roles related to the clinical setting • **Compare** roles and responsibilities of health care professionals across the organisation and **outline** how they relate, or differ • **Review** nursing bands and **compare** the different responsibilities between the bands, for trained and untrained nurses • **List** key people to contact in my service and **book** one-to-one meetings with them during my supernumerary time (check with my preceptor who to prioritise) • **Discuss** roles, and service priorities related to role, with the key people I meet • **Describe** how each role may affect patient care and the service

What is a SMART goal and how do I write them?

The widely used acronym SMART can help you set learning goals that can be measured, and their achievement will help show your progression and development in your role. SMART goals can be written in practice development plans to focus your learning and guide your future practice. SMART goals should be:

Specific, Measurable, Achievable, Realistic and Time-based

Details linked to each element of the acronym are presented in *Box 2.5*.

Box 2.5 Elements of the SMART acronym

Specific	• Goal is specific and significant to your learning and development • Goal is clear to understand, concise and well defined
Measurable	• Goal is quantifiable, to allow you to measure the outcome when completed • Goal has an established benchmark for measuring
Achievable	• Goal is achievable and accessible • Goal is based on your skill and resources • Goal is based in your area of practice • Goal is action-orientated, containing an action verb • Goals should be agreed between you and your preceptor
Realistic	• Goal should be realistic, relevant and applicable to your practice role • Goal should be achieved within available resources and time
Time-based	• Goal should have specific timelines attached along with a feasible deadline for completion of goals • There should be enough time to complete the goal

Example stages to help you write a SMART goal are presented in *Box 2.6*.

Box 2.6 Example stages to help develop and write a SMART goal

Stage 1 Start by just identifying what you want to learn:

"I want to learn about all the different nursing roles on my new ward."

Stage 2 Be specific and try to write it down in one sentence. Remember to be clear and concise and not use vague words like 'I want', as you will not know when you have reached your goal:

"To increase my understanding of different nursing roles and staff responsibilities on my new ward."

Stage 3 Use an action verb to describe what you want to achieve. This will make your goal measurable:

"To increase my understanding of different nursing roles and staff responsibilities on my ward, by identifying all relevant nursing roles and determining how each role is responsible for patient and service delivery on my ward."

Stage 4 Link the goal to your specific practice with timelines for achievement and completion:

"Within 1 month post-qualification, I will identify all relevant nursing roles within my ward area and determine the nursing responsibilities related to each role and the effect these roles have on patient care and service delivery."

Stage 5 Add how you will show you have completed the goal and then you have your SMART goal!

Once written, you can always check your goals – is the goal below **S**pecific, **M**easurable, **A**chievable, **R**ealistic and **T**ime-based?

SMART GOAL:

"Within 1 month post-qualification, my preceptor will assess that I have the required level of knowledge and understanding of all nursing roles and staff responsibilities within my ward, and the effect these roles have on patient care and delivery."

Professional development plan and 3-monthly reviews

During your career you will require regular development reviews, which should be structured using a professional development plan (PDP). Some areas call them a professional development review (PDR). During your preceptorship period you should ideally have a ***professional development review at 3, 6, 9 and 12 months post-qualification*** and a 12-month ***annual appraisal*** with your line manager. See *Box 2.7* for an example pathway for goals and PDRs during your first year qualified. The reviews are based on evaluating your learning goals, objectives or role-specific competencies and signing off their completion. Following your review, new goals will be set and a future date for review will be planned, ideally within 3–6 months. You should be able to discuss any specific learning needs and training opportunities during your review to help your future career progression.

Your line manager or preceptor should complete your professional reviews. Ideally, your line manager would be your preceptor, but if there are a high number of new starter nurses, and a shortage of senior nurses, this may not be feasible.

Additional handy tips

There are some additional tips to help you structure learning during your first few months qualified:

- **Meeting key health care professionals, networking and visiting departments** can increase your insights and quickly orientate you to an area. Never underestimate the power of a friendly introduction and becoming friends with an experienced ward clerk or nursing assistant. Their help may be invaluable when you are busy, e.g. booking hospital transport. Ask your preceptor to identify which department visits and key people should be prioritised during your first month qualified. Be sure to document who you have visited, their role and contact details, the date you visited them, and any notes you made at the visit/meeting.

- **Ask your local pharmacist for a list of key medications used in your clinical setting,** to help you identify key actions and side-effects before you start to administer medications to patients yourself. It will give you a head start before you are accountable for medicines management and your supernumerary time is discontinued, and will increase your confidence when explaining drug actions and side-effects to patients.

- **Read patient information leaflets from your clinical or community setting;** if you feel overwhelmed by the amount you need to know they will give you a simple overview of key conditions, anatomy and physiology; and treatments that you will regularly come across. This information will help you to educate patients about their condition, or the investigations and procedures that will be taking place.

Box 2.7 An example pathway for goals and development reviews during your first year qualified

1 month post-qualified

- Meet your line manager and/or preceptor within your first week

- Complete induction and statutory and mandatory training (check timelines for completion with your line manager)

- Identify how much supernumerary time you have and what is expected during this time

- Write learning goals and objectives to complete at 3 months post-qualification, within first few weeks with your preceptor

- Identify and complete any role-specific competencies/learning objectives/goals required within 1 month post-qualification

- Align your rota/shifts to an experienced shift buddy and your preceptor for at least the next 3 months, but preferably the first year post-qualified

- Complete your supernumerary period and orientation checklist

- By Month One agree aims, objectives and goals for the next 3 months with your preceptor/line manager

3 months post-qualified

- Complete band 5 competencies required at 3 months post-qualification

- Complete learning objectives and goals set for your 3-month review

- Meet preceptor for 3-month professional development review (PDR) and set goals for your 6-month review. It is helpful to bring personal reflections and feedback from others to all your review and preceptor feedback forms (*Box 2.1*)

6 months post-qualified

- Complete band 5 competencies, learning objectives and goals set for 6-month review
- Meet preceptor for 6-month PDR and set goals for 9-month review

9 months post-qualified

- Complete band 5 competencies, learning objectives and goals set for 9-month review
- Meet preceptor for 9-month PDR and set goals for 12-month review

12 months post-qualified

- Complete 12-month PDR of learning objectives and goals with preceptor and/or line manager
- During your review identify your learning needs, your key interests in nursing and any future opportunities for you to develop your career, e.g. band 6 role
- Complete appraisal with line manager and/or preceptor and set goals and objectives for year 2
- Discuss your future career plans and aspirations in your appraisal
- During your appraisal establish how you can be supported by your line manager to move your career forward

- **Talk to staff who are relatively new in your area,** as they may have good tips or learning aids that you can use. One of our new starters wrote a comprehensive list of abbreviations for medical terms, such as 'ABX = antibiotics'. She found abbreviations very confusing during patient handovers and decided to share her work with other new starters. These abbreviations are now embedded within new starter orientations. You may want to start identifying key abbreviations in your clinical setting too, if there are some you do not understand. The *Abbreviations* page at the start of this book may be helpful.

- **Try to keep in touch with nurses who qualified with you,** or other band 5 new starter nurses, as they will often be feeling the same nerves and dealing with the same challenges as you. They can relate to how you feel and give you a sense of context and offer support, as you share similar experiences.

- **Identify experienced and approachable staff for support early on,** to make sure that you are well supported during those initial months.

- **Try to be assertive without being too pushy, if you lack confidence.** Some newly qualified nurses I meet are reluctant to tell others how they feel when they first start in practice, in case they upset people who do not know them very well. In comparison, others may assert their views too strongly, whilst not taking account of the global view of a situation. Ask experienced nurses to guide you before you address an unfamiliar issue if you are unsure how to gauge a conversation/situation. A few practical tips on being assertive when you first start are shown below:

Active listening

- Always use active listening to try to understand the other person's view.

- Listening to the other person gives you more control, rather than reacting emotively to what they say.

- Pay attention to what the other person is saying, acknowledge their view and then inform them of your view, as it shows assertiveness and professionalism, e.g. *"I understand why you have told me to do this ....; however, I feel like this ...., and I need to make you aware of this ....".* You are taking control and saying how you feel whilst clearly asserting your views.

Open problem-solving

- If you do not share honest feelings with the person/group/team they will never know your real viewpoint and you will eventually become frustrated.

- Take a problem-solving approach to the situation and think about what you are trying to get across:
  - what is the specific issue?
  - why is it an issue for you?

- how has the issue made you feel/how has the situation affected you?
- what would you like to happen, to resolve the issue?
- how can this person/others help you?
- what will happen if the issue is resolved/not resolved?
- what are your options if you are not supported/listened to?
- write notes on the above to help keep you focused.

Prepare well and do your research

- Debates and arguments are usually won through an evidence-based viewpoint underpinned by facts. Obviously, being assertive is not just about *'winning arguments'* when you are trying to assert yourself but having clear factual information, timelines or documentation will help support your perspective.
- Practise being assertive if you have a particularly difficult situation to address and run through what you are going to say beforehand.
- Check if others are feeling the same and constructively try to sort out issues together as a team.

Promote positivity from the start

- Try to book a meeting with the person/group in a calm and quiet environment to prevent interruptions.
- Thank the person/people at the start of the conversation for meeting with you and *'for constructively helping me with an issue that I have'*.
- Starting a conversation in a positive manner is much better than breaking out into a rant. Even if the other person/people launch into a tirade it does not mean you have to. Listening to others venting their frustrations is a more powerful social position to hold than joining in and allows you time to plan an informed reply later.

Learn to compromise and see the wider picture

- As a student nurse you become used to pushing for your competencies to be signed off amid busy placements, as the focus is on your individual learning needs. In the work arena you are one of a number of employees, which means you need to develop patience and a global view of situations.

- It is easy to jump in and become angry when your needs are not met, without finding out the facts. You may be angry that your annual leave is not on the rota but before moaning at your line manager, try to find out why it was not granted. Did you adhere to the policy when requesting your leave or is it just a genuine mistake that your manager can quickly rectify?

- Sometimes two people have very different viewpoints and a compromise needs to be sought. Talk through issues with an experienced nurse in a confidential supervision session. Senior nurses and HR staff can also offer confidential mediation between staff members.

Avoid extreme reactions

- Always try to keep calm and professional.

- Avoid emotive accusations and aggressive language by keeping to the facts.

- Plan what you are going to say before an important conversation/meeting, as you are more likely to stick to the brief.

Take control if you feel uncomfortable

- Working in a pressurised work environment means that people sometimes become frustrated at a situation and take it out on the nearest person in the vicinity, so try not to take this personally.

- You have the right to take control of a situation that is making you feel uncomfortable, e.g. by stopping the conversation. Acknowledge that you can see the person is frustrated/angry and suggest that you continue the conversation later when the person has calmed down. You are taking control, not allowing them to continue to vent at you, setting clear boundaries and offering to resolve the situation at a later stage. This demonstrates a professional and assertive approach.

- If you feel yourself becoming frustrated, try to take time out to calm down.

- Remember, saying nothing is sometimes the best option, rather than saying something that you might regret later. You can always come back to an issue once you have had time to reflect on what has upset you and can call on experienced colleagues to guide/support you.

Identify your 'triggers' and weaknesses

- Difficult conversations and challenges cause stress, which is why people choose to avoid certain people and not assert themselves in a situation. It is important that you develop your self-awareness when dealing with difficult issues by requesting feedback from experienced nurses who have observed you dealing with challenges in practice (see further guidance on team working in *Section 5.3* and dealing with difficult situations in *Section 8.3*).

- The SCARF model (Rock, 2008) describes five circumstances that may 'trigger' a reaction in people, such as another person criticising you, uncertainty in relation to outcomes, not having control over a situation, feeling excluded and being treated unfairly. Increase your self-awareness by reflecting on what your 'triggers' or weaknesses are, to prevent you overreacting in the future.

Learn from your mistakes

- Being assertive is a skill that anyone can learn through watching others who do it really well, reflecting on your own experiences and receiving constructive feedback from others.

- Never beat yourself up about a situation you feel went badly, and talk to someone senior about how you feel. On occasion, we all have to deal with a person/situation we would rather avoid. Every senior nurse can recall dealing with a past issue they would rather forget.

Remember, it is those thousands of interactions you have during your career that build your resilience and skill set, to enable you to handle future situations and become a role model to others!

Finally, the tip I give to newly qualified nurses is:

> ❝ *Always ask experienced staff for help, no matter how trivial you think your question is. Questions are a sign of an inquiring mind and a safe nurse; they are not a sign of weakness!* ❞

REFERENCES

Department of Health (2010) *Preceptorship Framework for Newly Registered Nurses, Midwives and Allied Health Professionals.* London: The Stationery Office.

Nursing and Midwifery Council (2008) *Standards to Support Learning and Assessment in Practice: NMC standards for mentors, practice teachers and teachers.* Available at: www.nmc.org.uk/globalassets/ sitedocuments/standards/nmc-standards-to-support-learning-assessment.pdf (last accessed 10 June 2018)

Nursing and Midwifery Council (2018) *Future Nurse: standards of proficiency for registered nurses.* Available at: www.nmc.org.uk/ globalassets/sitedocuments/education-standards/future-nurse-proficiencies.pdf (last accessed 10 June 2018)

Rock, D. (2008) SCARF: a brain-based model for collaborating with and influencing others. *NeuroLeadership Journal,* **1**: 1–9.

WHAT TO DO NEXT

1. Identify what to expect during your first few months qualified and approach your learning in a structured and methodical way, to decrease your initial anxieties.

2. Identify what statutory and mandatory training you need to complete and determine when training must be completed as your first training priority.

3. Devise an orientation checklist, identifying key information required in practice, which will help focus your key learning when you start in post.

4. Ensure you have a 'buddy' on every shift during your orientation period to ensure you have a trained nurse to support you if you have any concerns.

5. Establish which assessment and review methods your clinical setting will use to support your development, e.g. band 5 role-specific competencies, learning objectives and SMART goals.

6. Proactively book your professional development reviews at 3, 6, 9 and 12 months post-qualification and your annual appraisal with your line manager at 12 months.

7. Identify your preceptor and find out what preceptorship will be offered during your first year qualified.

CHAPTER 3

UNDERSTANDING THE KEY STRUCTURES IN NURSING

&& *I wish I had understood nurses' banding better, and how banding relates to different nursing responsibilities. It is really important to know who to delegate to when you first start in post, and you need to know what nurses below a band 5 are allowed to do when you delegate care to them. Nursing Assistants have different titles in different areas, such as Clinical Support Workers, Health Care Workers and Health Care Assistants, which is confusing. They can also receive a variety of training according to their banding, which relates to their level of competence and core responsibilities in practice.* 55

1 year post-qualified adult nurse

&& *I had no idea that there were different nursing delivery systems that could be used in practice until I started my first post. The first ward I worked on when I qualified used primary nursing, and I had only ever worked in a team nursing system as a student nurse. I am about to move to my second post on a ward that uses an intentional rounding approach. It would have been really helpful to have had an overview of the differences between nursing organisational systems when I first qualified.* 55

2 years post-qualified ward nurse about to move to second post

When I support newly qualified nurses in practice they often want to know about the nursing structures in their working environment. Their requests usually relate to three key questions: "*What nursing structures and organisational systems do I need to learn about first?*", "*What do the different nursing titles and bands mean?*" and "*What is each nursing band accountable for?*". This chapter attempts to answer these questions, offering clear guidance as to the key structures you need to know about and the relevance they have to your role as a newly qualified nurse.

3.1 PAST STRUCTURES AND INFLUENCES ON TODAY'S HEALTH CARE

When I started my career as a nurse in the 1980s, NHS structures were very different from today. Health care funding was centralised and under the control of Regional Health Authorities. With the publication of the National Health Service and Community Care Act in 1990, NHS trusts were formed, and an 'internal market' was introduced (DH, 1990). The new internal market meant that health authorities stopped managing hospitals and had to 'purchase' care from hospitals instead. GPs also became 'fund holders', purchasing care for their patients, while the NHS trusts became 'providers' of care. The internal market encouraged competition but also increased local differences across the UK, which is sometimes referred to as a 'postcode lottery'. More recently, the 2012 Health and Social Care Act led to further NHS restructuring, and GP practices are now organised into wider clinical commissioning groups (CCGs) and primary care trusts (PCTs) and strategic health authorities (SHAs) were abolished (DH, 2012). Regular structural changes in the NHS will continue, as governments come and go. You should try to develop early in your career a basic understanding of how these NHS structures work, as future changes will inevitably influence the nursing care you deliver during your career.

In the 1980s, the majority of hospital and community settings were led by one sister/charge nurse (CN) and their deputy. The sister/CN accompanied consultants during their ward rounds, often starting with tea and biscuits in the consultant's office – hence the term 'doctor's handmaiden'. Only senior nurses had the keys to the drug cupboards and they administered all patients' medication on 'drug rounds'. As a new staff nurse, my main job was to act as a medication second checker, admit patients, write patient care plans, complete observations, and provide all other personal care for patients, delegated by the senior nurse. Only a matron would be able to administer intravenous (IV) drugs and senior nurses at the time were outraged that nurses were suddenly being asked to administer IVs, considering it to be purely a doctor's job.

Nursing roles were also less diverse, in contrast to the wide number of job titles and roles available today. It was standard for newly qualified nurses to begin as a staff nurse, progressing to a deputy sister/CN only after several years in their role. There were none of the link lecturer, clinical educator or practice development clinical nursing posts you find today. Apart from Macmillan nurses, specialist nurses and advanced nurse practitioners did not exist and only began to develop widely in the early 1990s.

The most prevalent nursing delivery system in the 1980s was 'task allocation'. This reflected the medical model, where the patient is viewed as a set of 'signs' and 'symptoms', and the nurse was given a series of 'tasks' on every shift from the nurse in charge. As a newly qualified nurse, I would be ordered to complete observational 'tasks', carrying out a temperature, pulse and blood pressure on each of our 28 ward patients. Under the task allocation system, patients were all woken up at 6am and had their breakfast before 8am; and the care delivered was rigid and less person-centred. Nurses today will still use a task allocation approach on occasion, when clinical settings are understaffed, or during emergencies, as it is still an efficient method to ensure numerous key tasks are completed in a timely manner whilst ensuring patient safety.

The 'named nurse' concept

Nursing moved towards a more patient-centred approach to care with the introduction of the 'named nurse' concept in the 1991 *Patient's Charter* (DH, 1991). The charter presented a series of rights for NHS patients that highlighted the importance of 'continuity of care' (see *Box 3.1*). Nursing professionals supported this patient-focused approach, which also resulted in the creation of many autonomous specialist nursing roles across all nursing fields.

> ### Box 3.1 The 'named nurse' concept
>
> *"The charter standard is that you shall have a named qualified nurse, midwife or health visitor who will be responsible for your nursing or midwifery care."*
>
> (Department of Health, 1991, p.15)

In 2013, the named nurse concept re-emerged, following one of the worst UK hospital scandals in recent years, which occurred in a district hospital in Stafford. 'Mid Staffs' became synonymous with negligent nursing care and high hospital mortality rates. The Mid Staffordshire NHS Foundation Trust Public Inquiry (Francis, 2013) ensued, and the government requested assurance that hospital nurses would provide a compassionate, patient-centred approach. As a result, all patients were to be given a 'named nurse and consultant', written above their hospital beds, to enable them to know who was responsible for their care.

The named nurse concept today is often synonymous with a primary nursing delivery system, due to its focus on continuity of care carried out by one registered nurse (see nursing delivery systems in *Section 3.3*). However, there are variable accounts of the feasibility of all patients having a named nurse in practice. Areas with high patient turnover, such as A&E and outpatients, or areas with high staff turnover that rely on agency nurses, may find it difficult to allocate a named nurse for the duration of a patient's stay. There is also a lack of professional prescription surrounding the named nurse concept and newly qualified nurses can, understandably, become confused about areas of accountability and responsibility, and the legal implications of being a named nurse today (see *Box 3.2*).

Box 3.2 Accountability and the named nurse

The named nurse

All registered nurses and midwives are responsible and accountable for providing continuous and consistent care using individualised care plans to meet patients' needs. It is generally agreed that the named nurse is one registered nurse, midwife or specialist community public health nurse who is accountable for the continuity of care of a particular patient from when they are admitted until they are discharged from a service. This does not mean the named nurse is legally responsible and accountable for that patient's care when they are off duty. If a nurse does not feel ready to become a named nurse for a particular patient, due to their lack of knowledge or experience, or the patient's complex needs, they should say so.

The senior nurse/midwife

The senior nurse/midwife is responsible for ensuring that the registered nurse or midwife is competent and capable enough to practise as a named nurse. If a registered nurse or midwife voices concern that they are not ready to be a named nurse for a particular patient, and the patient is subsequently negligently injured, then the senior nurse/midwife could be considered negligent due to unfair delegation.

When you arrive in your clinical or community setting, you should be told whether they support the named nurse concept and if so, you should ask the following questions:

- How is the named nurse documented, e.g. on admission documentation, above the patient's bed or in their care plan?
- How is the named nurse implemented in practice, e.g. does the patient receive information on the role of the named nurse?
- Does the practice area offer you specific advice/training on the named nurse role?
- How do they assess whether you are competent to be a named nurse?
- What happens when you are not on shift or unable to work in the community for a period of time, e.g. is the named nurse role allocated to another key person/worker?
- What happens if your patient deteriorates or you do not feel competent to care for the patient's needs without senior nurse support?

In contrast to the named nurse concept, your clinical area may offer a patient allocation or total patient care nursing delivery system, whereby nurses will be allocated to the patient on a shift by shift basis, or caseload basis in the community. Patient allocation and caseload management may be related to the geography of a clinical or community setting or patients' acuity (see *Chapter 4*). Your clinical setting may offer a mixture of both the named nurse and other delivery systems (see alternative nursing delivery systems in *Section 3.3*).

3.2 KEY LOCAL AND NATIONAL STRUCTURES

As a newly qualified nurse you do not work in isolation, and it is important that you have a basic knowledge of key national and local structures. These structures will include important people, and professional and legal governing institutions and bodies.

Local management structures

Whether you choose to work in the NHS or the private sector, it is helpful for you to know how your local organisational structures work. You may receive a diagram from your local HR department or line manager, with key trust departments and personnel detailed, and usually placed in order of responsibility.

NHS trusts are essentially public sector businesses and if you work on a ward/department in a trust you will see a board of directors, and executive and non-executive members, at the top of the organisation. It is a good idea to find out their names and what they look like, as they may visit your area to ask you questions about your work environment and the care you are providing (their photos are usually found on trust websites). Often key executive staff in trusts will hold information-sharing meetings, open to all employees, that will keep you updated on future strategic plans. These open forums are interesting to attend and give staff an opportunity to put forward their views.

The trust board of directors has overall responsibility for the trust strategy – for example, ensuring that trust activity meets demand, and that the trust keeps within financial budgets and meets all quality targets set by the government. The trust management executive is the senior managerial decision-making body and is usually chaired by the chief executive. The chief executive will be the person called to give interviews to the media if there are any local issues or new initiatives to promote. There is also a democratically elected council of governors who are unpaid members who hold the trust board to account. All trust boards are required to have an audit committee consisting only of non-executive directors.

Trust services will be split into clinical services that may be headed by a divisional director or general manager. It is helpful to find out how departments across your trust are structured and where your department sits, relative to other services. There will always be a head nurse in some capacity responsible for all nursing staff in an NHS trust; they are sometimes called a lead nurse, director of nursing, chief nurse or clinical nurse director. There should be a clearly defined nursing structure under the head nurse in your trust and it is helpful to know who your senior nurses are, such as your divisional nurse or matron/assistant matron.

Private sector employers, such as a nursing home, are not bound by standard NHS structures as they are privately owned businesses. A typical private nursing home will be headed by a director of operations who makes sure that the overall business goals are met. In a large nursing home there may be a number of assistant directors. The director of operations is usually the face of the nursing home and in charge of administration. They have a key role in obtaining external funding from sponsors and marketing their service, and they are not involved in the day-to-day care of patients. The majority of nursing homes employ a chief nursing officer (they may have a different title) who manages all the employees who deliver direct care, and they work collaboratively with the director of operations. The chief nursing officer's main responsibility is to ensure that all nursing care standards are maintained. In contrast to a chief nursing officer, nurse managers in nursing homes are responsible for a smaller number of staff and residents, and they report to the chief nursing officer.

Private hospitals often have a similar structure to nursing homes in relation to operational management; however, ratios of trained to untrained nurses are different, as nursing homes usually use a higher ratio of nursing assistants. Private hospitals often have the same senior nursing structures as NHS hospitals, e.g. matron, sister/CN and deputies.

Structures in community care settings were changed in 2013, following the creation of clinical commissioning groups (CCGs) that replaced primary care trusts (PCTs). CCGs are clinically led statutory bodies responsible for the planning and commissioning of health services for a local area. The CCGs are structured as membership bodies with local GP practices as members. They are controlled by an elected governing body made up of GPs and other clinicians, which should include a lay member, registered nurse and secondary care consultant. CCGs are responsible for commissioning mental health services, emergency care, rehabilitation care, elective hospital services and community care. The CCGs are answerable to the Secretary of State for Health through NHS England. Although there is a collaborative 'group' structure evident within CCGs, there are clearly defined national nursing structures in the community for district nursing and general practice nurses. Band 8 advanced community nurse practitioners and senior district nurses/team leaders at band 7 would be responsible for service development, maintaining standards and delegating responsibilities and caseloads to a nursing team, covering a defined locality or practice population.

National structures

Key national professional and legal governing institutions/bodies are presented in *Table 3.1*.

Table 3.1: Key national institutions and bodies

National institution / body	Role	Key responsibilities
The Department of Health (DH)	Ministerial department responsible for government policy on health and social care	Overseeing the National Health Service (NHS)
		Providing strategic leadership and funding for the NHS, public health and social care
		Developing and creating national policies and guidelines to improve the quality of care, meet health care demands and patients' expectations
		Providing long-term vision to address future health care challenges
		Assuring the delivery of services and their continuity
		Representing the best interests of the public, patient and taxpayer
The Secretary of State for Health	Government cabinet minister with responsibility for the work of the DH	Responsibility for health in the NHS, which includes the policies of the department, financial control, performance and delivery, and patient safety
NHS England / Scotland / Wales / Northern Ireland	Executive non-departmental public body of the DH	Setting the priorities and direction in the NHS to improve health care outcomes for people
		Focusing on the operational side and delivery of commissioning in the NHS
Public Health England (PHE) / NHS Health Scotland / Public Health Wales	Executive agency of the DH	Providing national leadership and expert services to support public health
		Working with local government and the NHS to respond to emergencies
		Providing education for the public to make healthier choices
		Addressing health care inequalities

Care Quality Commission (CQC)	Executive non-departmental public body of the DH	Independently regulating and inspecting health and social care services in England
		Assuring that health care services in England provide people with safe and effective care
		Encouraging care services to improve through carrying out inspections and monitoring data that can indicate problems
		Registering care providers and rating services
		Taking action to protect patients who use services and protecting the rights of vulnerable people
The Nursing and Midwifery Council (NMC)	Statutory regulating professional body for nursing and midwifery professionals in the UK	Maintaining a national register of all nurses, midwives and specialist community public health nurses eligible to practise within the UK
		Protecting the public by setting standards of nurse education, training, conduct and performance
		Investigating allegations of incompetence and impaired fitness to practise
The National Institute for Health and Care Excellence (NICE)	Executive non-departmental public body of the DH in the UK	Providing a national evidence base to guide improvements to health for the public and patients (originally set up to end the 'postcode lottery')
		Providing information and developing quality standards for those commissioning health, public health and social care services
		Appraising the use of health technologies, treatments and procedures within the NHS to guide practice on appropriate treatment

(continued)

Table 3.1: (Continued)

National institution / body	Role	Key responsibilities
The Royal College of Nursing (RCN)	Professional membership organisation and trade union for nurses and midwives in the UK	Promoting excellence in practice and shaping UK health policies
		Representing the professional interests of nursing staff working in the public, private and voluntary sectors
		Lobbying UK institutions and bodies to influence policies to improve quality patient care
		Supporting and approving nursing standards, education and practice
		Hosting a specialist nursing library (the largest in Europe)
		Providing courses for nurses in their Royal College of Nursing Institute
		Collaborating with key UK bodies to negotiate pay and terms and conditions, for public and independent sector nurses

3.3 KEY TYPES OF NURSING DELIVERY SYSTEMS

Nursing care delivery systems are theoretical or philosophical frameworks that describe how nurses should approach and deliver patient care. These delivery systems provide a method to allocate nurses to patients and influence the patient care approach, in a clinical or community setting. Nursing delivery systems used across health care services can vary greatly and may be embedded adhering to their true principles, or changed according to circumstances, such as a lack of staff and increase in patient acuity.

Historically, nursing delivery systems are divided into four types:

- **Task allocation**
- **Primary nursing**
- **Team nursing**
- **Patient allocation.**

Total patient care is also a method of organising patient care that allocates one practitioner to carry out all the patient's care requirements. It is often used in intensive care settings, in home care settings or when students have one or two patients to care for.

Intentional rounding involves nurses carrying out regular checks on patients using a scripted approach to ensure their fundamental care needs are met. This approach gained attention in 2006, following a US study by Meade *et al.* (2006) that measured the effect of using a checklist approach during hourly intentional rounds on call bell use, patient satisfaction and safety. In the UK, intentional rounding was lauded as a way to promote regular interactions at the bedside following the Mid Staffordshire NHS Foundation Trust Public Inquiry (Francis, 2013).

An overview of key nursing delivery systems is presented in *Table 3.2*, which includes the principles, advantages and disadvantages of each system.

3.4 THE DIFFERENCES BETWEEN NURSING ROLES AND BANDS

Four key areas of nursing

Due to the diverse nature of nursing today, and the lack of standardisation of roles across the UK, you may become confused by the different job titles. Most nursing roles relate to one of four key areas:

Table 3.2: Overview of key nursing delivery systems

Key principles and methods	Potential advantages and disadvantages
Task allocation	
Nurse in charge of a shift assigns different tasks to specific nurses based on the patient's care plans	**Advantages**
	Can be used intermittently during shifts under any nursing system during a crisis
Assignment of care links to 'tasks' rather than patients, e.g. emptying all urinary catheters on a ward	Allows urgent tasks to be completed quickly to ensure patient safety and can be appropriate to use during staff shortages
Autocratic approach where decisions are made by the nurse in charge, who decides which tasks are completed by whom during the shift	Allows appropriate skills to be assigned to nursing assistants (NAs) and complex tasks to registered nurses
	Rules and rituals can promote a consistent approach
Communication is hierarchical	Junior staff stress is reduced as problems addressed by senior nurses
	Economic and efficient care can be assured
	Disadvantages
	Lacks an individualised approach as routines become task-orientated
	Does not reflect humanistic model
	Focuses on physical care
	Patient confused by different nurses
	Care fragmented and does not reflect holism
Team nursing	
Team leader allocates patients to team members during a shift	**Advantages**
	Team members deliver patient care that increases staff satisfaction
Patient assignment based on the level of experience of team members, patient acuity and tasks to be completed during a shift	Patient care delivered through coordination and cooperation between team members
	Reduces fragmented care
Communication hierarchical as all staff must report to the team leader / nurse in charge	NAs and students feel well supported and part of a team
Patients are assigned and delegated according to each team member's level of responsibility and accountability	Stress and fatigue less as workload can be coordinated and shared
	Team members utilise their skills according to their expertise

Table 3.2: *(Continued)*

Key principles and methods	Potential advantages and disadvantages
	Disadvantages
	Not all teams work well as a group
	Relies on good leadership
	Time required coordinating the team
	If team leader a poor communicator this will negatively impact on the delivery of care
	If team membership is not consistent it leads to a decrease in patient satisfaction
	Responsibilities become fragmented without good leadership
	Time required to know the level of competence of team members before allocation

Primary nursing

Registered primary nurse is assigned to a patient from admission to discharge, to ensure continuity of care	**Advantages**
	Continuity of care achieved with a defined primary nurse for every patient
Primary nurse leads patient care and directs other team members and colleagues	Supports collaborative and interdisciplinary care
	Useful in hospice or nursing home setting to aid continuity of care
Primary nurse accepts responsibility and accountability for decisions made with team support	Improved patient–nurse relationship
If a primary nurse is not available, an associate nurse is responsible for patient care during their absence	**Disadvantages**
	Difficult to deliver if high turnover of staff/patients or increased patient acuity levels
	Dependent on the quality of staff knowledge and experience
	If patients' needs are challenging it can increase stress on the primary nurse

Patient allocation

Patient allocation is delegated over a single shift by a registered nurse/nurse in charge	**Advantages**
	Communication is direct and patients usually allocated after a nursing handover
Patients allocated will vary from shift to shift, based on geography and patient acuity	Nurses are able to negotiate the patients/workloads given to them

(continued)

Table 3.2: (Continued)

Key principles and methods	Potential advantages and disadvantages
Different methods are used to allocate caseloads according to patients' needs and staff experience	Increases staff involvement in the delivery of care
	Promotes nurses' decision-making
	Often allocations linked to geographic closeness that aids communication across large areas
	Disadvantages
	Disagreement about allocations between staff
	Poor communication / personality clashes in teams can lead to inappropriate allocations / caseloads
	Poor leadership and inexperienced nurses can lead to inappropriate allocation / caseloads
	Each nurse may have a different approach to care
	Allocation may cover too long distances

Intentional rounding

Nurses carry out 1–2-hourly checks on the patient to ensure their fundamental care needs are met during the shift	**Advantages**
	Increases patient satisfaction due to the regular presence of a nurse over a shift
Nurses use scripts and a checklist approach to care throughout the shift, using a mnemonic, e.g. the **4 Ps** – **P**ositioning, **P**ersonal needs, **P**ain and **P**lacement	Improves staff responsiveness to meet patients' needs during rounding over a shift
	Patients benefit from regular communication with their nurse at the bedside
Anticipates and delivers fundamental care rather than responding to call bells	Positive effect on patient outcomes such as a reduction in falls, pressure ulcers, patient complaints and call bell use, and an increase in patient satisfaction
'Intention' and actions performed during rounds on a shift are associated with an aspect of patient care that can be measured	Assures managers that patients will not be left unattended for long
	Disadvantages
	Staff not carrying out checks properly and turning rounding into a tick box approach
	May not be suitable for rehabilitation areas, or for less mobile / cognitively aware patients
	High patient acuity levels can cause a lack of rounds
	Shown to be unsuccessful if staff are unmotivated or not engaged in the process
	Viewed by some as a top-down management approach that is autocratic
	The 'needs' aspect and use of mnemonics reflects a task-based approach

- Clinical
- Specialist
- Research
- Education.

Some example UK nursing roles are presented under each of the four areas in *Box 3.3*. Nursing roles may also cross over areas, having a mixture of responsibilities, for example my lecturer practitioner role is split as 50% education and 50% clinical. What encompasses 'clinical' in a role may range from 'hands-on' patient care delivering all fundamental care needs, to managing a large number of clinical staff with minimal direct 'hands-on' care.

Box 3.3 Jobs and nursing areas

Nursing area	Example nursing job titles
Clinical	Staff nurse, sister/charge nurse (CN), deputy sister/CN, registered staff nurse, team leader, clinical lead, lead practitioner, senior nurse, clinical services manager, matron, nurse consultant, non-medical prescriber, head of care, head of care and quality, clinical governance practitioner
Education	Practice development nurse, clinical nurse educator, clinical educator, education lead, nurse educator, practice nurse educator, education facilitator, lecturer practitioner, practice supervisor, practice assessor, academic assessor
Specialist	Specialist practitioner, specialist nurse, specialist nurse practitioner, advanced nurse practitioner, senior advanced nurse practitioner
Research	Research nurse, research practitioner, specialist research nurse

Differences between nursing bands 2–4

As a newly qualified nurse, you will have worked with numerous unregistered nurses as part of your training and gained some insights into these roles. When you first qualify, however, it is important to have an overview of which band 2–4 nursing roles are actually utilised within your setting. It is essential that you understand the banding, qualifications and competence levels relating to these roles, as you will be delegating care to these members of staff. Checking the generic job descriptions of nurses in bands 2–4 in your area is a helpful way to give you a general insight into the differences between bands, along with an explanation from your line manager or preceptor.

Band 2 nurses are usually called a nursing assistant (NA), clinical support worker (CSW), support worker (SW) or health care assistant (HCA). Band 2 nurses work under the direct supervision of the registered nurse and are responsible for supporting registered nurses to deliver routine care to patients.

Band 3 nurses are usually **senior NAs, CSWs, SWs or HCAs**. There is a great disparity between roles and expectations of band 3 nurses across the UK, as there is no current national standard or registration of the role. It is widely acknowledged that a band 3 nurse should take on advanced skills relating to additional training they have received, such as a level 3 National Vocational Qualification (NVQ) or a national Care Certificate. The Care Certificate consists of fifteen standards of learning outcomes and competencies expected of a nursing assistant. A band 3 nurse should also actively contribute to care planning by liaising with the registered nurse, taking on additional link roles in the setting, or supporting junior band 2s.

Band 4 nurses are called **nursing associates** and the NMC plans to open up a new part of the NMC register for nursing associates in 2019. Some band 4s are called assistant practitioners (**APs**) but it is expected that all future band 4 roles will align with the new **nursing associate** title and proficiencies.

Band 4 nurses have a higher level of knowledge and skill than band 2 or 3 nurses, and they deliver elements of clinical work that have previously been within the remit of registered nurses, such as:

- Performing patient assessments from admission to discharge and writing patient care plans
- Recording and interpreting observations and escalating concerns
- Assessing and monitoring patients' skin integrity and reporting/documenting changes
- Recognising changes in a patient's condition and reporting to a registered nurse/medic

- Performing, understanding and reporting patient risk assessments
- Actively participating in handover to ensure continuity of care
- Using equipment and medical devices (following appropriate training)
- Engaging in reflective practice
- Demonstrating understanding of informed consent, the Mental Capacity Act and Deprivation of Liberty, and applying these principles to their care.

In April 2018, the NMC produced draft *Standards of Proficiency for Nursing Associates* (NMC, 2018a) for consultation; these are mapped against the latest *Standards of Proficiency for Registered Nurses* (NMC, 2018b). The aim of these proficiencies is to explicitly demonstrate the differences between a band 4 and band 5 role. Nursing associate proficiencies are structured under six headings, as opposed to the new registered nursing proficiencies, structured under *'seven platforms'*.

Following this national consultation, the expectation is that future band 4 nursing associates will be professionally accountable to administer certain medications and to undertake drug calculations for a range of medicines (NMC, 2018a). It is evident that registered nurse proficiencies are set to a higher level than associate nurse ones, in key areas such as primary assessment, developing care plans, overseeing and monitoring care, working in teams, coordinating/delegating care, and improving the safety and quality of care (NMC, 2018b).

The band 4 role is relatively new to the NHS and requires a higher level of education to a foundation degree level in health and social care, or equivalent. The band 4 nurse works alongside band 2/3 nurses and registered nurses to deliver fundamental care within their scope of practice, which is defined by employers within their job description and person specification. It is important that you keep up to date with future changes relating to nursing roles within your profession. When you start in practice it is useful to check the local job descriptions, competence levels and skills of band 4s and band 3s working in your area to compare the differences.

Differences between nursing bands 5–9

Whatever your chosen field, you will work in a team of registered nurses who will range in banding from 5 upwards. Specific job descriptions and person specifications will give you information about registered nursing roles in your area. Typical generic differences in roles and responsibilities between bands 5 to 9 are shown below:

Band 5

- Delivers high quality patient care adhering to national and local, legal and professional requirements
- Delivers care for a named group of patients
- Responsible for own caseload under indirect supervision of senior nurse
- Professionally accountable for assessing, planning, implementing and evaluating patient care, using patient care plans and the Nursing Process
- Teaches students and unregistered nurses
- Practice supervisor for students
- Works collaboratively with MDT to facilitate effective patient care
- Promotes patient wellbeing through education and health promotion
- Provides family-centred care and support for relatives/carers
- Oversees and monitors patient care
- Works in teams, coordinating and delegating care
- Improves the safety of patients
- Improves the quality of patient care.

Band 6

- Responsible for delivering patient-focused care (as band 5) whilst also influencing the delivery of care by others in their team, e.g. supporting a team of colleagues
- Responsible for supporting the senior nurse to assist with managing, developing and leading the service (deputises for senior nurse)
- Acts as a professional role model
- Contributes to the provision and maintenance of high standards in the clinical setting
- Uses initiative to organise and prioritise workloads of others, e.g. shift coordinator or monitoring standards
- Responsible for inducting/supporting/developing a group of staff

- Practice supervisor for students
- Practice assessor for students.

Band 7

- Responsible for delivering high standards of patient care across their service (as above)
- Provides clinical leadership and management of a nursing ward team/service
- Effectively supports band 8
- Responsible for the day-to-day management of a ward/service and provides effective management of resources
- Budget holding for staff and services
- Responsible for maintaining compliance with professional and legal standards and targets, whether national and local
- Ensures adherence to local and national policies and guidelines.

Band 8

- Strategically plans clinical services
- Responsible for day-to-day organisation and delivery in clinical departments/settings to meet local and national targets
- Supports initiatives within the service whilst providing clear direction for staff
- Responsible for deployment, motivation, development and performance of all clinical staff across their services
- Ensures the achievement of CQC standards.

(Nurse consultants and educational leads at band 8 will have similar responsibilities linked to educational or patient care pathway targets.)

Band 9

- Directs services, and manages and leads all nursing bands (8 and below) within their service
- Reports to the managing director to develop and implement changes within a strategic framework
- Ensures financial targets are achieved across all services

- Responsible for developing the strategic vision and transformation plans in the local health care system
- Ensures operational and clinical services are delivered and quality is assured
- Responsible for assuring safe and effective patient-centred care is delivered
- Provides detailed analysis of the sustainability of future services
- Promotes innovations that can enhance the service.

Future restructuring

Having experienced numerous changes to the structuring of nursing during my 30-year career, I can safely say that you too can expect many changes in the future. The restructuring of health care services and nursing responsibilities will inevitably continue in order to meet the ever-growing needs of our ageing and increasing population. The digital era will increase the use of information technology across health care, and more complex interventions will in the future be delivered in homes and GP surgeries, rather than hospitals. It is important, therefore, that you are aware of the current structures within your chosen profession, whilst also informing yourself of any future plans to restructure. My key advice to all newly qualified nurses:

> **"** You have many more opportunities today to influence the progression and restructuring of nursing through research than any nurses have ever had in the past. With the theory and knowledge generated from nursing research comes the power to influence your future profession, working environments, staffing levels and nursing structures. Without nursing research you will continue to have others telling you how to structure and organise the delivery of future nursing care. **"**

REFERENCES

Department of Health (1990) *National Health Service and Community Care Act.* London: The Stationery Office.

Department of Health (1991) *The Patient's Charter.* London: The Stationery Office.

Department of Health (2012) *The Health and Social Care Act.* London: The Stationery Office.

Francis, R. (2013) *Report of the Mid Staffordshire NHS Foundation Trust Public Inquiry: Executive Summary.* London: The Stationery Office.

Meade, C.M., Bursell, A.L. and Ketelsen, L. (2006) Effects on nursing rounds: on patients' call light use, satisfaction, and safety. *American Journal of Nursing,* **106**(9): 58–70.

Nursing and Midwifery Council (2018a) *Standards of Proficiency for Nursing Associates (DRAFT – April 2018).* Available at: www.nmc. org.uk/globalassets/sitedocuments/na-consultation/standards-of-proficiency-for-nursing-associates.pdf (last accessed 10 June 2018)

Nursing and Midwifery Council (2018b) *Future Nurse: standards of proficiency for registered nurses.* Available at: www.nmc.org. uk/globalassets/sitedocuments/education-standards/future-nurse-proficiencies.pdf (last accessed 10 June 2018)

WHAT TO DO NEXT
---

1. Establish a basic understanding of how NHS structures work nationally and within your local area.

2. Find out how your area supports the 'named nurse' concept and what you are expected to deliver in practice.

3. Find out what nursing delivery systems are used in your area and how they are implemented in practice.

4. Check the generic roles and job descriptions of a band 2 to 9 in your setting to gain an understanding of the differences between bands.

5. Establish what band 2–4 nurses in your area are competent to do, before you delegate care to them.

6. Check local job descriptions, competence levels and skills of a band 4 and band 3 working in your area to compare the differences.

7. Keep up to date with changes to professional standards and nursing roles in the future.

CHAPTER 4

UNDERSTANDING SAFE STAFFING AND PATIENT ACUITY AND DEPENDENCY TOOLS

66 *When I qualified, I wish I had understood how senior nurses organised staffing across wards. I remember one of my shifts where I panicked as my ward buddy had gone to theatre. I ended up being the most senior nurse with two other health care assistants. We were looking after lots of dependent patients and I didn't know where to start. Luckily, the senior nurse who was coordinating the floor happened to walk onto the ward. She literally started helping me take patients to the toilet and told me to always ring the floor coordinator if I needed extra support in the future. She stayed with me until the nurse in charge came back. I now make sure that all our new starters know there is always someone senior on another ward, or at the end of a phone, whatever time of day or night, and they are never alone.* 99

1 year post-qualified adult nurse

66 *I had no idea there were ways of allocating patients to staff at the beginning of shifts using acuity and dependency scores. I also didn't know what the sister meant by calling me a 'whole time equivalent' when she was sorting out my rota. I found out that using acuity and dependency scores at the start of your shift helped spread the workload across the team and stopped one nurse from being overloaded. It's important to know about these tools, even if your practice area doesn't use them. One of the nurses I shared a house with showed me the dependency scoring tool used on her ward. I decided to show my ward sister and asked if I could evaluate the tool over a month to see if it would help with our workloads. I had recently been appointed*

as a practice educator so it fitted with my new role. After our evaluation, we are going to introduce acuity and dependency scores into every handover to help with patient allocation on a shift by shift basis. **"**

16 months post-qualified practice educator

When I support newly qualified nurses in practice, they often worry about safe staffing and how they should organise their care if patient acuity and dependency are high across their working environment. Their requests usually relate to the following questions: *"What are safe staffing levels and how do we know we are safely staffed?"*, *"What do the different acuity and dependency scoring systems mean?"* and *"What do I do if I feel the staffing levels are unsafe in my practice area?"*. This chapter attempts to answer these questions, offering clear guidance relating to safe staffing; it also covers patient acuity and dependency scores and how to deal with future staffing issues, should they arise.

4.1 PAST METHODS USED TO DETERMINE STAFFING LEVELS FOR NURSES

When I worked as a junior staff nurse in the 1980s, the sister would allocate a number of patients to every nurse on the shift after the handover. The allocation of patients was usually according to patients' geographic location and nurses' experience.

There were no computers in practice and everything was written on paper or verbally handed over. This important handover detailed particularly dependent patients, the number of trained/untrained nurses and additional issues predicted for the next shift. Having reviewed every ward handover, the nursing officer had an overview of what was happening across the hospital and would decide where a *'pool'* of extra nurses would be sent. Every hospital and community setting had a pool of NHS-employed nurses who were financed centrally and worked in any area requiring extra help. In the 1980s NHS staffing budgets were centralised and set for periods of 12–14 years by health authorities, which made these additional nurses easier to finance.

In contrast to the 1980s, today's nurse staffing budgets are set annually and may change if overspend occurs during the financial year. Nursing employers tend to request additional nurses from local agencies, and senior nurses have to check their staffing budgets according to set parameters, prior to requesting additional staff.

Early patient classification systems

In the 1980s, patient classification systems started to emerge to guide nurse staffing levels, according to a patient's stage of illness and their capacity to function in daily life.

Initial classifications attempted to measure the severity of an illness and its effects on the patient using:

- a **disease-orientated approach** based on diagnosis, clinical findings, stages of illness or treatments
- a **function-orientated approach** based on severity/limitations of an illness on the individual's normal life.

Early patient classification systems relied on nurses' expertise and individual decision-making. They acknowledged that senior nurses had the knowledge to decide their own staffing levels; they were, however, subjective and open to human error. Local systems varied across hospitals and they were not used to evaluate staffing costs relating to the delivery of care. In the late 1980s, there was a dramatic increase in NHS expenditure, which led to a focus on the costs of *'operational services'* and the *'delivery of resources'*. Staffing data started to reflect the characteristics of the clinical setting such as nursing expertise, skill mix and study for education, and nursing delivery systems, such as team nursing.

4.2 TODAY'S NHS

Today's NHS strives for clinical services to be efficient and cost-effective. The amount and intensity of workload for a nurse continues to increase across clinical and community settings. Health care employers are, therefore, using empirical approaches to set and monitor nurse staffing parameters. Theory-based systems decrease subjective decision-making and promote cost-effective standardisation to meet increasing service demands. Current and future service pressures include:

- The number of NHS hospital beds in the UK (including learning disability, maternity, acute/general, mental illness and day beds) has halved over the past 30 years, whilst numbers of patients admitted has significantly increased (King's Fund, 2017).
- A current, and predicted, rise in an ageing UK population:
  - the number of people aged 65 or over in the UK is expected to rise by 40% in the next 17 years

- by 2040, one in four people in the UK will be 65 or over
- the number of people over 85 in the UK is predicted to double in the next 23 years to over 3.4 million (Office for National Statistics, 2017)

- Increasing demand for UK nursing care homes
- Earlier discharge of patients with more complex medical problems
- Global research developing treatments requiring more expensive interventions.

Nurse staffing levels are affected by increasing service demands and budgets. They are also influenced by the number of student nurses trained and the retention of current workforces. As a newly qualified nurse, try to keep up to date with national and local staffing guidance, which may lead to changes in staffing levels within your profession. When you start as a newly qualified nurse, it is important that you have a basic understanding of how your local service is staffed, and what the agreed safe staffing levels/ratios are.

4.3 IMPORTANT SAFE STAFFING GUIDANCE FOR NURSES

Key terms

It is helpful for you to gain an understanding of the key terms relating to nurse staffing, patient acuity and dependency.

Nurse staffing

- This term refers to the size and skill mix of your nursing team and needs to be placed in context with your local area.
- It is usually expressed as nursing care hours for each nurse (per patient per shift) or total nursing hours (across a setting over a 24-hour period).

Nursing skill mix

- This relates to the grouping together of different categories of nurses and is an essential part of workforce planning.
- It is determined by ratios, numbers or percentage of types of nurses within a team; for example, ratios of registered nurse to health care assistant, numbers or percentages of bands of nurses.

Safe nurse staffing

Safe nurse staffing requires:

- satisfactory numbers of nurses, measured according to nurse : patient ratios
- satisfactory skill mix, measured according to RN : HCA ratios
- nurses with essential skills
- lead nurses who organise appropriately.

Professional bodies, such as the Royal College of Nursing (RCN), provide guidance on minimum essential safe staffing levels that are evidence-based. Currently, there is no government legislation on minimum safe nurse staffing levels.

Patient acuity and dependency

- Acuity and dependency 'scores' quantify the level of reliance a patient has on assisted care from an RN.
- The higher the score, the more dependent/acute the patient is.
- There is evidence of specific acuity/dependency tools being used widely across services.
- Patient acuity/dependency scores can be used as a reference for estimating nurse staffing levels, establishment and staffing budgets.

Nursing establishment

- The total number and type or band of nurses working across your clinical area or community setting is called the *nursing establishment.*
- Managers aim to keep their nursing establishment within their allocated staff budget using a mix of nursing bands.
- Employers usually plan nursing establishments in advance of a financial year.

Caseload

- The term *'caseload'* refers to the care of groups of patients over a given time period (it applies to hospital caseloads and community-based caseloads).
- Caseloads include family and carer support and reflect the acuity/dependency of the groups of patients you are caring for.

- If you are a district nurse your caseload may reflect a geographical area or be aligned to a general practice.
- District nurses' caseloads vary in size, and workload will depend on:
  - individual needs of patients
  - demographic profile of the population covered
  - geographical distribution of patients.

Bed occupancy

Bed occupancy is the number of patients in a hospital ward, unit or community hospital, expressed as a percentage. For example, 100% *bed occupancy*, during the period April 2016 to April 2017, on a ward means no bed was left empty (unoccupied) without a patient in it during this annual period.

WTE (whole time equivalent)

Whole time equivalent is a common term used to express nursing establishments in real terms by taking account of full- and part-time staff.

- 1 nurse working full-time (FT) 37.5 hours per week is classed as 1.0 WTE.
- 1 nurse working half a week part-time hours (PT) = 18.75 hrs per week = 0.5 WTE.
- 2 nurses working PT 18.75 hours per week each = 1.0 WTE.

Planned staffing hours

Planned staffing hours denotes the amount of hours staff are expected to work, based on an approved template.

Actual hours

Actual hours is the amount of hours actually worked by staff, which will take into account sickness, maternity leave and compassionate leave.

Live staffing data

- Most nursing rotas are available on an electronic roster system that will contain *live staffing data*.

- Live staffing data allows you to find out how many hours you have worked over the course of a month, or are owing, and how much annual leave you have left.

- You can gain access to your rotas and live staffing data through your line manager.

What you need to know about safe staffing levels for nurses

In 2011, the Royal College of Nursing (RCN) voted in favour of legally enforced nurse staffing levels at their RCN congress, in order to safeguard patient care (RCN, 2011). Since this significant vote, there has been no UK government legislation for **minimum nurse staffing levels or trained : untrained staffing ratios**, using validated tools.

In April 2018, however, Wales became the first country in Europe to legislate nurse staffing levels, following the passing of the Nurse Staffing Levels (Wales) Act 2016 (National Assembly for Wales, 2016). Under this new legislation, NHS employers in Wales must calculate the number of nurses they require and ensure that *'they are making efforts to maintain staffing levels'* in adult acute medical and surgical inpatient areas. Although the Nurse Staffing Levels (Wales) Act 2016 does not mandate minimum staffing levels or staffing ratios, it places an obligation on health boards to calculate, and take steps to maintain, safe nurse staffing levels. NHS Wales supports the use of the *Welsh Levels of Care* reference document (NHS Wales, 2017) that uses a triangulated approach to guide the assignment of acuity descriptor levels to aid staffing calculations (see the section on specific workplace planning tools in *Section 4.4*). The *Welsh Levels of Care* document is used by nurses to substantiate their professional judgement about their patients' levels of acuity and staffing requirements.

UK nurse staffing levels, and skill mix ratios between RNs and support workers, continue to be agreed at local level. There is, however, evidence of a centralised approach to workforce planning through the use of mandated tools across Scotland and Wales. Nationally determined ranges (not ratios) of *'staff : beds'* are used in Northern Ireland. In comparison, a number of English university hospitals are using consistent evidence-based tools to determine optimal staffing levels. Perspectives on workforce planning from the different countries comprising the UK are shown below.

England

- **Department of Health England** does not standardise the approach to nurse staffing.

- Each ward determines its own nurse staffing requirements; however, there are groups of English university hospitals using evidence-based tools, such as the Safer Nursing Care Tool, to determine optimal staffing levels (Shelford Group, 2013).

- The Care Hours per Patient Day (CHPPD) measure is also recommended by the Department of Health as a consistent way of recording nursing staff required over 24-hour periods in English adult inpatient hospital wards.

- CHPPD measures can inform nursing establishments and operational plans across NHS trusts (Carter, 2016).

Northern Ireland

- **The Department of Health, Social Services and Public Safety (DHSSPS) in Northern Ireland** promotes the use of nationally determined normative ranges using a framework of *'nurse : bed'* ranges (DHSSPS, 2014).

- Nurse : bed ranges are **triangulated** with the Telford (1979) method to determine nursing establishments, to determine types and numbers of nurses required.

- There is limited evidence of how many areas use the DHSSPS (2014), as the framework is not nationally mandated.

Scotland

- **NHS Scotland** established a collection of twelve field-specific Nursing and Midwifery Workforce and Workload Planning tools for local use.

- Data from tools informs nurse staffing levels when triangulated with clinical outcome data and expert judgement (NHS Scotland, 2017).

- The majority of Scottish health care providers use the nationally mandated tools to inform nurse staffing levels.

- The Scottish government is aiming to legislate on the use of mandated workforce planning tools by all NHS providers across Scotland.

Wales

- **The Nurse Staffing Levels (Wales) Act 2016** (National Assembly for Wales, 2016) came into force in April 2018. NHS employers in Wales must calculate the numbers of nurses they need and ensure they are making efforts to maintain safe staffing levels. The Act does not mandate on minimum staff : patient ratios.

- **NHS Wales** approved the implementation of the Welsh Level of Care workforce tool that uses a triangulated approach to support professional judgements made by nurses relating to patients' acuity levels and nurse staffing requirements.

Interestingly, there are regions in **other countries that have legislated** and implemented minimum mandatory nurse : patient ratios; see *Table 4.1*.

Table 4.1: Legislated nurse : patient ratios in some other countries

Country	Clinical setting	RN : patient ratios
California, USA (CNA and NNOC, 2008)	Medical / surgery wards	1 RN : 5 patients
	Mental health inpatient	1 RN : 6 patients
	Paediatrics	1 RN : 4 patients
	Antepartum	1 RN : 4 patients
New South Wales, Australia (NSWNA, 2011)	Medical / surgery wards	1 RN : 4 patients
	Palliative care wards	1 RN : 4 patients
	Mental health inpatient	1 RN : 4 patients
Victoria, Australia (DHHS, State Government of Victoria, Australia, 2015)	Acute general and medical surgical wards	1 RN : 4 patients

Monitoring nurse staffing levels

English nursing employers must ensure they have adequate staffing levels to meet the standard required, during any Care Quality Commission (CQC) inspection. Inspectors examine whether an employer has sufficient numbers of 'skilled' nursing staff to deliver safe care. In Scotland, the equivalent inspection body is Healthcare Improvement Scotland; in Wales it is Healthcare Inspectorate Wales. In Northern Ireland the equivalent inspection body is the Regulation and Quality Improvement Authority.

Senior nurses aim to maintain their nursing numbers and skill mix according to predetermined levels agreed by their employers, e.g. the NHS trust, clinical commissioning group or private institution. **Staffing numbers and skill mix ratios should not be viewed in isolation, and staffing tools should be triangulated with patient acuity / dependency scores, to establish an accurate picture of nursing workforce demands.** On a hospital ward, for example, you could have ten patients who are low dependency and waiting to be discharged, or four immobile patients with tracheostomies who each need regular 1:1 care. The nurse with four patients would have a much higher dependency and workload than the nurse with ten patients. Extra patient dependency information will therefore give you a more accurate view of workload demands, as opposed to purely RN : HCA numbers and skill mix ratios.

Current staffing recommendations for nurses

Key professional bodies, such as the RCN, offer clear recommendations for UK nurse staffing levels and skill mix ratios, to guide nurse employers. These professional bodies also recommend the additional use of acuity and dependency tools, or workforce planning tools, to establish optimal staffing levels. Using recommended triangulated approaches enables employers to establish what constitutes 'safe', 'unsafe' or 'at risk' staffing across local areas. Some examples of nurse staffing ratios and skill mix percentage, which are recommended by professional bodies, are summarised in *Table 4.2*. To gain an accurate representation of staffing requirements, and optimal staffing levels in your practice area, check on staffing parameters with your line manager.

Safe nursing indicators (SNIs)

Nursing staff are able to request assistance with their staffing levels at any time, to maintain standards of patient care, if they risk falling to 'at risk' or 'unsafe' levels. However, if a senior nurse requests to close beds, authorisation is usually sought from their employer. The decision to authorise bed closures, or request additional staff, is balanced between the need to stay financially afloat and maintain safe staffing levels, the latter being the main priority. Employers continually monitor their ability to hit key targets, to avoid being financially penalised, and share staffing across services if required. Millions of pounds in funding are withheld from NHS providers every financial year due to fines imposed for breaching key performance targets, such as the 18-week target for non-urgent operations and 4-hour waiting times in A&E. Many hospital and community settings have daily bed meetings and caseload reviews, to enable them to keep their services working at full capacity. If you have an opportunity to attend such meetings, try to observe the tools used to maintain safe staffing levels, move staff and authorise bed closures.

Senior nurses usually provide evidence of SNIs not being met, prior to bed closures or booking extra staff outside staffing budgets (NICE, 2015). Examples of SNIs, and the ways in which they can be measured, include:

Official complaints

- **Complaints:** linked to nursing and care staff
- Friends and family response rates.

Safety outcome measures

- **Falls:** the severity of falls, e.g. no harm/moderate harm/death.
- **Pressure ulcers:** hospital-/institution-acquired pressure ulcers (category 2, 3 or 4)
- **Increase in harm:** adverse events or mortality rates, patients acquiring MRSA (methicillin-resistant *Staphylococcus aureus*), *Clostridium difficile*
- **Call bells:** percentage of call bells answered within 5 minutes (target 95%).

Staff reported measures

Staff breaks: Percentage of missed breaks, percentage of breaks not taken over time, percentage of extra hours worked.

Ward nursing establishment measures

- **Staffing:** planned, required, and available nursing staff for each shift indicates staffing *'at risk'* or *'unsafe'*
- **High reliance on extra staff,** e.g. bank or agency staff
- **Lack of staff compliance** with mandatory training.

It is important that you are aware of SNIs to inform any future escalation of staffing issues, if indicated. As an RN, you should officially report any SNIs you come across in practice, according to local escalation and incident reporting policies.

Table 4.2: UK nurse staffing recommendations from key professional bodies

UK speciality	Professional body	Recommendations (minimum recommendations only and staffing levels will also depend on the specialist needs of patients at the time)
Adult intensive care unit (ICU)	British Association of Critical Care Nurses (BACCN) (2009)	1 RN : 1 ventilated patient
		Each ICU patient to have access to 1 RN with post-registration qualification
		1 supernumerary senior critical care qualified to units of 6 beds or more
		RN : patient ratio on adult ICU should not fall below 1 RN : 2 patients
General paediatric wards	RCN (2003)	Under 2 years = 1 RN : 3 children
		Above 2 years = 1 RN : 4 children (day shift)
	RCN (2013) (revised additions)	Revised: above 2 years = 1 RN : 4 children (day and night shift)
		Minimum skill mix RN : support worker = 70:30 (varies according to specialist need, e.g. ICU has higher ratio of trained staff)
		Shift supernumerary supervisor in each clinical area to ensure effective management and supervision of staff
		Specialist nurses and advanced nurse practitioners not to be included in bedside establishments
		At least 1 nurse per shift will be trained in the Advanced Paediatric Life Support (APLS) course / European Paediatric Life Support (EPLS) course (depends on service needs)
		Minimum of 2 registered children's nurses at all times in inpatient and day units
		70% of nurses should have specific training required for the speciality, e.g. children's oncology
		Patient dependency scoring should be used to provide an evidence base to adjust staffing levels daily
		There should be access to a senior children's nurse for advice at all times

Neonatal services	RCN (2013)	1 RN : 4 neonatal special care infants 1 RN : 2 high dependency infants 1 RN : 1 intensive care infant
Midwifery	NICE (2015)	More than 1 registered midwife (RM) : 1 woman in established labour 1 RM : 1 woman throughout the whole of labour; not necessarily the same RM Other staffing ratios for other stages of labour developed locally
	Ball *et al.* (2014)	Skill mix RM : MSW (midwife support worker) = 90:10 96 birth cases per WTE RM in community (not involving actual birth)
Children's intensive care and high dependency	PICS (2015)	0.5 RN : 1 patient (children requiring close supervision and post-op monitoring) 1 RN : 1 patient (child nursed in cubicle, with a mental health problem requiring close supervision or a deteriorating condition requiring ICU) 1 nurse with appropriate level competences in paediatric critical care : 1 child needing level 3 critical care
Acute mental health ward	Royal College of Psychiatrists (2010)	A ward of 15 acute patients would be unsafe with fewer than 3 RNs per shift during the day and 2 RNs at night (Note: higher staffing levels may be essential if patient is acutely ill, requiring 1:1 care)
Mental health services	NHS England (2015b)	Lack of benchmarking specific to mental health staffing requirements Use mental health staffing framework for support that is not prescriptive (currently recommends 2 workforce calculator tools tests)

(continued)

Table 4.2: (Continued)

UK speciality	Professional body	Recommendations (minimum recommendations only and staffing levels will also depend on the specialist needs of patients at the time)
Nursing homes in Northern Ireland	Regulation and Quality Improvement Authority (RQIA) (2009) in Northern Ireland	1 RN : 5 patients (early shift) 1 RN : 6 patients (late shift) 1 RN : 10 patients (night shift) Skill mix RN : health care assistant (HCA) = 35:65 for all shifts **(Note: RN : HCA ratios are opposite to those recommended for the older person by the RCN (2012) below)**
Older people's wards	RCN (2012)	Skill mix RN : HCA = 75:35 for good quality care for the older person Skill mix RN : HCA = 50:50 for basic care 1 RN : 5 patients and never exceeding 1 RN : 7 patients
Acute general and surgical wards in England	RCN (2006) and RCN (2012)	Skill mix RN : HCA 65:35
General and specialist medical and surgical wards adult in-hospital care in Northern Ireland	DHSSPS Northern Ireland (2014)	Framework uses *nurse : bed* ranges along with Telford's (1979) method of determining establishments: • General medicine 1 RN : 1.3–1.4 beds • Specialist medicine 1 RN : 1.4–1.8 beds • General surgery 1 RN : 1.25–1.4 beds • Specialist surgery 1 RN : 1.4–1.8 beds

Adult inpatient wards in acute hospitals	NICE (2014)	No single staff : patient ratio can be applied across all adult inpatient wards
		If RN caring for more than 8 patients during a day shift, closely monitor for evidence of increased harm and nursing red flag events
District and community nursing	NHS Improvement (2016)	Acknowledges lack of evidence and research, recommends the following:
		• Development of a national classification system for nurse staffing in the community
		• Economic analysis to understand effectiveness of district community nursing services
		• Development of national markers and metrics as indicators of sufficient workforce, and use of staffing tools that currently exist
		• Evidence-based processes for workforce planning at a local level
	Queen's Nursing Institute (2016)	Advocates using the term *'safe caseloads'* as opposed to *'safe staffing'* to reflect a *'whole approach'* in community settings
	NHS England (2015a)	District community nurses must have appropriate skills and competence to deliver quality care and have time for supervision of complex caseloads

NOTE: *Professional recommendations may change from the time of publication and you may have local differences, according to specialisms/numbers of beds/caseloads/geographical locations. Please check local staffing guidance and policy with your line manager.*

Publishing staffing information

In June 2014, it became a national requirement for all hospitals to publish information about nurse staffing levels on wards, including the number of shifts meeting agreed levels (NICE, 2014; DH, 2014). This was in response to recommendations from two widely publicised public inquiries that investigated claims of patient abuse and neglect:

- The Winterbourne View Hospital public inquiry (DH, 2012)
- The Mid Staffordshire NHS Foundation Trust public inquiry (Francis, 2013)

In 2014, NHS England and the Care Quality Commission issued joint guidance to trusts on the delivery of the 'Hard Truths' commitments (NHS England, 2014), requesting the publication of nurse staffing data that included the following:

- Staff numbers (planned numbers and actual numbers) displayed on boards outside all inpatient ward areas.
- Trusts displaying and evaluating staffing data and publishing reports online (safer staffing data is published monthly on NHS Choices, via UNIFY reporting, and the public can view data in one place).
- Six-monthly trust board report detailing the *'capacity'* and *'capability'* of wards (monthly reporting relates to planned versus actual staffing and includes staffing vacancies. Trusts must complete a 6-month review of their nurse staffing establishments for external publication (DH, 2014).

As a newly qualified nurse, it may be helpful for you to view the above staffing establishment data, prior to deciding where you wish to start your career, or whilst you are working as a newly qualified nurse.

4.4 WORKFORCE PLANNING AND ACUITY AND DEPENDENCY TOOLS

A number of nursing workforce planning methods have been reviewed and tested by Hurst (2003), and his classification of approaches is widely used as a reference point throughout the UK today (see *Table 4.3* for a summary of approaches).

Specific workforce planning tools

NICE (2014) recommends that each ward determines their own staffing needs using acuity/dependency systems to aid decision-making. As a newly

Table 4.3: Types of workforce planning methods, how they work, and their strengths and weaknesses (adapted from Hurst, 2003)

Professional judgement approach (Telford, 1979)

Estimates number of working hours needed for each skill mix Calculations determine the available nurses per shift from a ward's nursing establishment Uses an expert group (clinical, workforce and finance) to estimate and decide the size and skill mix of each ward's team	**Strengths** Quick and easy method, good inexpensive starting point for managers Can be applied to any speciality Good foundation to use with complex methods
	Weaknesses Too subjective Association between staffing and nursing quality hard to explain Inflexible to changing patient numbers, acuities and dependencies

Nurses per occupied bed (NPOB) method

NPOB (known as 'top-down' method) Uses average numbers and ratios of nurses per occupied beds to determine staffing establishments	**Strengths** Quick and easy method Creates empirical data across nursing establishments, e.g. bed occupancy and skill mix ratios that can be divided into bands Used to benchmark across services
	Weaknesses No consideration of acuity and dependency Assumes baselines determined rationally Routinely collected data may be inaccurate

Acuity–quality method

Estimates and evaluates the size and mix of ward nursing teams using *'dependency–activity–quality'* or *'acuity–quality'* methods Obtains average numbers of patients in each dependency category and records the average amount of direct care time given to each dependency category per day Converts time differences into staffing activity / dependency ratios	**Strengths** Useful in wards where patient numbers and skill mix fluctuate Formulas are sensitive to the number and mix of patients in a ward (software packages available) Establishes standard below which nursing care should not fall Overcomes weaknesses in professional judgement / NPOB methods

(continued)

Table 4.3: *(Continued)*

	Weaknesses
	Formulas complex to create and manage
	Analysis of data requires computer spreadsheets
	Reflects nursing workload in high patient throughput wards better than on short stay units, such as outpatients or theatre departments
	Adds to nurses' workload

Timed-task/activity approach

Type and frequency of nursing interventions required by patients used as guide to staffing	**Strengths**
	Used when *acuity–quality* staffing methods are poor staffing predictors
Value (minutes) attached to each nursing intervention (reflects care plan) and amount of time to care for one patient over a 24-hour period is determined	Suits wards where care plans are systematically used and patients' needs can be predicted
	Patients' direct care needs are recorded locally
Patient's care plan updated each day and total hours for all patients generated by all care plans in the ward are combined	Easily computerised as part of a nursing information system
	Patient variables impacting on nursing time are considered
Wards' nursing hours are collected and validity checks completed by experienced staff to ensure consistency in recording nursing interventions	**Weaknesses**
	Effort needed to regularly update care plans
	Aligned commercial systems are expensive
	Some nurses disagree with quantifying individualised nursing care interventions

Regression-based system

Predicts required number of nurses for a given level of activity	**Strengths**
	Useful when predictions are possible, such as the number of planned admissions
The predictor is called the independent variable and the outcome (or level of staff) is known as the dependent variable	Helps managers plan for additional service demands
	Data easy and cheap to collect
Identifies an independent variable, e.g. acuity–quality data, to predict the number of staff (dependent variable)	Can compare across similar specialities
	Outcomes of regression models validated by other methods
	Weaknesses
	Statistician required to examine and analyse the regression data collected
	Wards providing data for regression analysis are assumed to operate efficiently
	Managers imposing regression techniques on teams alienate nurses who may feel they lack ownership

qualified nurse, it is helpful to know which specific workforce planning and acuity/dependency tools are used by your employer.

The 'Care Hours per Patient Day' (CHPPD) method: the Carter Report (Carter, 2016)

- This is a unit of measure to quantify nursing staff required and staff available in relation to the number of patients (can be condensed into nursing bands).
- It is only for use in hospital ward settings.
- It provides a consistent way to record and report deployment of staff on patient wards.
- It is calculated by adding the hours of RNs to the hours of HCAs and dividing the total by every 24 hours of inpatient admissions at midnight:

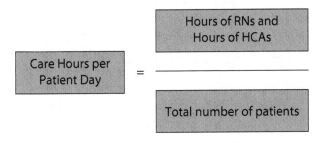

AUKUH Acuity/Dependency tool (the Association of UK University Hospitals (AUKUH), 2007)

- This classifies levels of patient care based on the Comprehensive Critical Care Classification (DH, 2000), levels 0–3, to determine level of acuity/dependency of all patients.
- The total acuity/dependency number of all patients is aligned to an evidence-based multiplier that recommends the level of nurse staffing required.
- Nurse sensitive indicators (NSIs) monitored and aligned to staffing levels.
- Example AUKUH (2007) scores (extracts only):
  - **Level 0:** patient's needs can be met through normal care, e.g. patient awaiting discharge

- Level 1: patient can be managed on inpatient ward; requires more than baseline resources
- Level 1a: acutely ill patient requiring intervention, or unstable with a greater potential to deteriorate
- Level 1b: patients who are in a stable condition but have increased dependence on nursing support
- Level 2: patients who are unstable and at risk of deteriorating and should not be cared for in general wards
- Level 3: patients needing advanced respiratory support and therapeutic support of multiple organs.

The Safer Nursing Care Tool (Shelford Group 2007) also endorsed by NICE (2014)

- This tool was developed by the Shelford Group (2007), consisting of ten leading NHS teaching hospitals.
- It is an evidence-based measure of patient acuity/dependency, used to calculate staffing levels for adult inpatient wards.
- The senior nurse assigns a dependency score to each patient each day and enters the score on an iPad, e.g. 12 patients at Level 0, 7 patients at Level 1a.
- Components of the tool include:
  - an acuity and dependency tool (AUKUH, 2007)
  - multipliers to calculate total staff needed in a particular ward
  - NSIs as quality indicators.
- The tool allows comparison across wards/trusts to ensure optimal staffing levels are benchmarked against agreed national standards.
- Measures are actual and not predictive.
- It is not suitable for small wards.

The Welsh Levels of Care (NHS Wales, 2017)

- A triangulated methodology is used to estimate the amount of nursing time required.
- The tool was developed by the All Wales Nurse Staffing Programme: NHS Wales, for adult acute medical and surgical inpatient areas.

- Welsh health boards/trusts are required to calculate the number and skill mix of nursing staff required to meet the needs of patients. That includes:
  - patient acuity levels
  - quality indicators
  - professional judgement.
- The Welsh Levels of Care (NHS Wales, 2017) consist of five levels of acuity:
  - **Level 1:** patient's condition is stable and predictable, requires only routine nursing care
  - **Level 2:** patient has a clearly defined problem but there may be a small number of additional factors that affect how treatment is provided
  - **Level 3:** patient may have a number of problems, some of which interact, making it more difficult to predict the outcome of any individual treatment
  - **Level 4:** patient is in a highly unstable and unpredictable condition, either related to their primary problem or an exacerbation of other related factors
  - **Level 5:** patient is highly unstable and at risk, and requires continuous 1:1 nursing care.
- The Welsh Levels of Care provide different types of descriptors to allow nurses flexibility when making judgements:
  - lay descriptors – describe the typical condition of a patient/types of care
  - clinical descriptors – detail professional considerations for each level
  - nursing themes – provide technical detail about conditions/interventions for each level.

Field-specific tools

Midwifery

Birthrate Plus is an established national software tool used to calculate midwifery staffing levels based on the *timed-task/activity* approach (Hurst, 2003; Ball *et al.*, 2014). Developed in the 1990s and endorsed by NICE, it is applied across the majority of NHS trusts in the UK and has been further developed over the years to reflect fluctuating working patterns. Required staffing and workforce establishments are calculated based on specific activity, case mix, demographics and skill mix.

Children's

The Great Ormond Street Hospital (GOSH) Paediatric Acuity and Nursing Dependency Assessment tool (PANDA) is an established national software tool developed to measure paediatric acuity and dependency, leading to a calculation of nursing requirements.

Community

There are no nationally validated tools to specifically calculate the number of community and district nurses required in an area; this is due to the dynamic nature of populations and individualised care required. Population size, age profiles and geography are currently used to determine staff capacity and skill mix in teams, judged on an individual basis.

As part of the Carter Review (DH, 2017), NHS Improvement is currently reviewing community and mental health care trusts to identify an 'optimal model' for staffing and is due to publish findings in the near future (DH, 2017).

What to do if you have staffing concerns

Research from the RN4CAST Nurse Survey in England has shown that staffing levels may impact on the quality of care and mortality rates. For example, higher HCA : bed ratios increase mortality rates by 5.4%, and there is a 7% decrease in likelihood of death related to a 10% increase in RNs (National Nursing Research Unit, 2012).

When you are newly qualified, spend some time establishing the following baseline data in your practice area:

Baseline staffing information

- Shift patterns and numbers of nurses (includes bands) on each shift
- Skill mix ratios of RN : support worker
- Senior nurse support on shifts (band 6 and 7)
- Process in place to ensure staffing establishments are met on a shift-to-shift basis

- Employer parameters set for safe staffing
- Dependency and acuity tools used
- Safe nursing indicators (SNIs) (see above)
- The rostering system in place, e.g. e-rostering.

Once you have a staffing baseline, check escalation policies and how to access senior nurse support if you are concerned about staffing at any time. Managers are responsible for routinely monitoring shift-to-shift staffing and delivering staffing solutions.

If staffing shortages are identified:

1. Establish the deficit of staff, e.g. numbers of staff or deficit in your skill mix.

2. Evidence the impact of this deficit on patient care (refer to information above on NSIs if indicated).

3. Initially escalate concerns to the nurse in charge, documenting the time and date in case there are complaints made later.

4. The nurse in charge should support you and reconfigure staffing on the shift, for example by asking team members to work with you or other patients. It is their responsibility to address staffing, on a shift-by-shift basis, and to support you. Future rotas should be reviewed and staff may be asked to arrive at work earlier.

5. The nurse in charge may escalate and request further assistance from their senior, if indicated. As a junior nurse, your role is to escalate to the immediate nurse in charge; however, if you are the most senior nurse at that time, you need to be aware of the local escalation policy to escalate urgent staffing matters to senior nurses.

6. You should be aware of the escalation policies in place and report where you think staffing capacity and capability falls short of what is required. Report any SNIs on an incident form and keep a record of who you escalated staffing concerns to.

7. Escalation policies outline:
   - actions to be taken
   - the people who should be involved in decisions relating to short-, medium- and long-term staffing shortages
   - the contingency steps where staffing problems cannot be resolved locally.

The escalation policy allows employers to adopt a proactive, rather than a reactive approach to staffing problems.

> 66 *Remember, never worry about asking for help as you are not alone and workload should be shared across your team. It is better to let senior nurses know you are concerned or struggling, to prevent future complaints and poor care.* 99

REFERENCES

Association of UK University Hospitals (2007) *Patient Care Portfolio: AUKUH Acuity and Dependency Tool. Implementation Resource Pack*. London: AUKUH.

Ball, J.A, Washbrook, M. and the Royal College of Midwives (2014) *Birthrate Plus: what it is and why you should be using it*. Available at: www.rcm.org.uk/sites/default/files/Birthrate%20Plus%20Report%20 12pp%20Feb%202014_3.pdf (last accessed 10 July 2018)

British Association of Critical Care Nurses (2009) *Standards for Nurse Staffing in Critical Care*. Newcastle upon Tyne: BACCN.

California Nurses Association (CNA) and National Nurses Organizing Committee (NNOC) (2008) *The Ratio Solution*. Oakland, CA: California Nurses Association. Available at https://nurses.3cdn.net/ cd91f6731ee0c22b41_uqm6yx8dy.pdf (last accessed 10 July 2018)

Carter, P.R. (2016) *Operational Productivity and Performance in English NHS Acute Hospitals: unwarranted variations*. London: Department of Health. Available at: www.gov.uk/government/uploads/system/ uploads/attachment_data/file/499229/Operational_productivity_A. pdf (last accessed 10 July 2018)

Department of Health (2000) *Comprehensive Critical Care: a review of adult critical care services*. London: The Stationery Office. Available at: http://webarchive.nationalarchives.gov.uk/20121014090959/http:// www.dh.gov.uk/prod_consum_dh/groups/dh_digitalassets/@dh/@en/ documents/digitalasset/dh_4082872.pdf (last accessed 10 July 2018)

Department of Health (2012) *Transforming care: a national response to Winterbourne View Hospital*. Department of Health Review: Final Report. London: The Stationery Office. Available at: https:// assets.publishing.service.gov.uk/government/uploads/system/uploads/ attachment_data/file/213215/final-report.pdf (last accessed 10 July 2018)

Department of Health (2014) *Hard Truths: the journey to putting patients first.* Volume One of the Government Response to the Mid Staffordshire NHS Foundation Trust Public Inquiry. London: The Stationery Office. Available at: www.gov.uk/government/uploads/system/uploads/attachment_data/file/270368/34658_Cm_8777_Vol_1_accessible.pdf (last accessed 10 July 2018)

Department of Health and Human Services, State Government of Victoria, Australia (2015) *Safe Patient Care (Nurse to Patient and Midwife to Patient Ratios) Act 2015.* Available at: www2.health.vic.gov.au/health-workforce/nursing-and-midwifery/safe-patient-care-act (last accessed 10 July 2018)

Department of Health, Social Services and Public Safety (2014) *Delivering Care: Nurse Staffing in Northern Ireland. Section 2: Using the Framework for general and specialist medical and surgical adult in-hospital care settings.* Belfast: DHSSPS. Available at: www.health-ni.gov.uk/sites/default/files/publications/dhssps/normative-staffing-ranges-section2.pdf (last accessed 10 July 2018)

Francis, R. (2013) *Report of the Mid Staffordshire NHS Foundation Trust Public Inquiry.* London: The Stationery Office. Available at: www.gov.uk/government/publications/report-of-the-mid-staffordshire-nhs-foundation-trust-public-inquiry (last accessed 10 July 2018)

Great Ormond Street Paediatric Acuity and Nursing Dependency Assessment tool (PANDA). Available at: www.gosh.nhs.uk/about-us/our-corporate-information/publications-and-reports/safe-nurse-staffing-report/gosh-panda-tool (accessed 10 July 2018)

Hurst, K. (2003) *Selecting and Applying Methods for Estimating the Size and Mix of Nursing Teams – A Systematic Review commissioned by the Department of Health.* Leeds: Nuffield Institute for Health. Available at http://www.who.int/hrh/tools/size_mix.pdf (last accessed 10 July 2018)

King's Fund (2017) *NHS Hospital Bed Numbers: past, present, future.* Available at: www.kingsfund.org.uk/publications/nhs-hospital-bed-numbers (last accessed 10 July 2018)

National Assembly for Wales (2016) Nurse Staffing Levels (Wales) Act 2016. Available at: www.legislation.gov.uk/anaw/2016/5/pdfs/anaw_20160005_en.pdf (last accessed 10 July 2018)

National Institute for Health and Care Excellence (2014) *Safe Staffing for Nursing in Adult Inpatient Wards in Acute Hospitals*. Guideline (SG1), published July 2014. Available at: www.nice.org.uk/guidance/sg1 (last accessed 10 July 2018)

National Institute for Health and Care Excellence (2015) *Safe Midwifery Staffing for Maternity Settings*. Guideline (NG4), published February 2015. Available at: www.nice.org.uk/guidance/ng4/resources/safe-midwifery-staffing-for-maternity-settings-pdf-51040125637 (last accessed 10 July 2018)

National Nursing Research Unit (2012) *RN4CAST Nurse Survey in England*. London: National Nursing Research Unit. Available at: www.kcl.ac.uk/nursing/research/nnru/publications/Reports/RN4Cast-Nurse-survey-report-27-6-12-FINAL.pdf (last accessed 10 July 2018)

New South Wales Nurses' Association (2011) The offer on ratios. *The Lamp*, **68(1)**: 16–17.

NHS England (2014) *Guidance Issued on Hard Truths Commitments Regarding the Publishing of Staffing Data*. Available at: www.england.nhs.uk/2014/04/hard-truths/ (last accessed 10 July 2018)

NHS England (2015a) *Framework for Commissioning Community Nursing*. Available at: www.england.nhs.uk/wp-content/uploads/2015/10/Framework-for-commissioning-community-nursing.pdf (last accessed 10 July 2018)

NHS England (2015b) *Mental Health Staffing Framework*. Available at: www.england.nhs.uk/6cs/wp-content/uploads/sites/25/2015/06/mh-staffing-v4.pdf (last accessed 10 July 2018)

NHS Improvement (2016) *Safe Caseloads for Adult Community Nursing Services: an updated review of the evidence*. Canterbury Christ Church University. Available at: https://create.canterbury.ac.uk/15373/1/Final%20Version%20Managing%20Safe%20Caseloads%20in%20Adult%20Community%20Nursing%20Settings%20with%20ISBN.pdf (last accessed 10 July 2018)

NHS Scotland (2017) *Nursing & Midwifery Workload and Workforce Planning Programme*. Available at: www.isdscotland.org/Health-Topics/Workforce/Nursing-and-Midwifery/NMWWP (last accessed 10 July 2018)

NHS Wales (2017) *Welsh Levels of Care (Edition 1)*. Cardiff: All Wales Nurse Staffing Programme. Available at: www.1000livesplus.wales.

nhs.uk/sitesplus/documents/1011/Published%20Welsh%20Levels%20 of%20Care%20%20edition%201.%20English%20version..pdf (last accessed 10 July 2018)

Office for National Statistics (2017) *UK Labour Market Statistics: Feb 2017.* Available at: www.ons.gov.uk/releases/uklabourmarket statisticsfeb2017 (last accessed 10 July 2018)

Paediatric Intensive Care Society (2015) *Quality Standards for the Care of Critically Ill Children* (5th edition). London: PICS. Available at http:// picsociety.uk/wp-content/uploads/2016/05/PICS_standards_2015.pdf (last accessed 10 July 2018)

Queen's Nursing Institute (2016). *Understanding Safe Caseloads in the District Nursing Service.* London: Queen's Nursing Institute. Available at: www.qni.org.uk/wp-content/uploads/2017/02/Understanding_ Safe_Caseloads_in_District_Nursing_Service_V1.0.pdf (last accessed 10 July 2018)

Regulation and Quality Improvement Authority (2009) *Staffing Guidance for Nursing Homes.* Belfast: RQIA.

Royal College of Nursing (2003) *Defining Staffing Levels for Children's and Young People's Services.* London: RCN.

Royal College of Nursing (2006) *Setting Appropriate Ward Nurse Staffing Levels in NHS Acute Trusts.* London: RCN.

Royal College of Nursing (2011) *Views from the Frontline – RCN Employment Survey.* London: RCN.

Royal College of Nursing (2012) *Safe Staffing for Older People's Wards.* London: RCN.

Royal College of Nursing (2013) *Defining Staffing Levels for Children's and Young People's Services.* London: RCN.

Royal College of Psychiatrists (2010) *Quality Standards for Liaison Psychiatry Services* (2nd edition). London: RCP.

Shelford Group (2013) *Safer Nursing Care Tool Implementation Resource Pack.* The Shelford Group/The Association of UK University Hospitals. Available at: http://shelfordgroup.org/library/documents/130719_Shelford _Safer_Nursing_FINAL.pdf (last accessed 20 August 2018)

Telford, W.A. (1979) A method of determining nursing establishments. *The Hospital and Health Services Review,* **5**(4): 11–17.

WHAT TO DO NEXT

1. Gain an accurate baseline of staffing requirements and optimal staffing levels in your practice area.

2. Identify safe staffing parameters with your line manager, e.g. agreed safe staffing ratios and numbers that will help inform any future escalation to senior nurses.

3. Identify which safe staffing workforce planning methods and acuity/dependency tools are used in your area. Identify what responsibilities you have regarding the recording and monitoring of regular data.

4. Review safe nursing indicators (SNIs) and officially report any SNIs you come across in practice, according to local escalation and incident reporting policies.

5. Review local escalation policy linked to reporting SNIs and unsafe staffing.

CHAPTER 5

PRIORITISING CARE AND DELEGATING TO OTHERS

ᴳᴳ *The one thing I worried about when I qualified was taking my own caseload, as I wasn't a student any more and my mentor wasn't there. I needn't have worried, as I was supernumerary alongside my team leader for 3 weeks. I realised from her feedback how much I did know from my nurse training. It is not just about having positive feedback though, as you need guidance on how to improve your time-keeping. I tended to focus on documentation too much, especially at the end of the shift, as I worried about missing important details. My team leader taught me how to develop my writing style to be more concise and factual; and to complete my documentation throughout the shift. If she had not pointed this out, I would still be going home late, writing pages of unnecessary description on my care plans.* ᴶᴶ

1 year post-qualified adult nurse

ᴳᴳ *I found delegating to clinical support workers really hard. I am naturally shy and wanted to look after the children allocated to me on a shift myself, just to make sure everything was completed correctly. I soon learnt that no nurse can do it all themselves on a busy ward, you have to learn to delegate! It is really helpful to find out what levels of HCAs you have on your ward when you start. I also found it helpful to watch our HCAs caring for the children I was looking after, to check what they were particularly good at.* ᴶᴶ

10 months post-qualified children's nurse

When newly qualified nurses begin their first shifts, they are faced with the responsibility of being accountable, as a 'named nurse' for a group of ward patients or for a caseload of patients across a community setting. The questions I am most frequently asked by new starter nurses during this period include: *"What is the best way to prioritise all the patients' needs when I have a group of patients to look after?"*, *"How do I delegate to other staff and manage a whole caseload?"*, *"Are there strategies I can use to help me prioritise my care and delegate to others?"* and *"How do I fit in with my new team?"*. This chapter attempts to answer these questions, offering clear guidance and practical examples to help you prioritise care, use appropriate delegation and successfully integrate into your new team.

When you start in practice, you will usually be part of a local team that directly delivers care, which is led by a corporate, or management/ hierarchical team structure. There will also be a multidisciplinary team (MDT) and/or interdisciplinary team (IDT) aligned to your practice area. The terms MDT and IDT are sometimes used interchangeably and/or incorrectly. The key differences between MDTs and IDTs are simply presented in *Table 5.1*.

Table 5.1: Differences between a multidisciplinary team and an interdisciplinary team

	Multidisciplinary team	Interdisciplinary team
Assessments	Assessments conducted by each discipline independently	Shared assessments and documentation
Professional boundaries	Clear set roles in the team according to professional boundaries	Professional boundaries may be blurred and professionals multi-skill
Communication	Professional communication takes place within each discipline	Professional communication takes place across all disciplines, usually through case conferences or case reviews
Record-keeping	Records are documented by each team member for individual patients	Records are shared with all team members through the use of integrated care pathways
Patient goals	Goals set within each discipline	All team members work towards shared patient-centred goals

5.1 SUPPORT IN PRACTICE TO DEVELOP YOUR MANAGEMENT AND LEADERSHIP SKILLS

Ever since Florence Nightingale established the first training school for nurses in 1860, registered nurses have had to make important decisions about what to prioritise, when caring for groups of patients, and how best to delegate to others in challenging environments. Out of all the chapters I am writing in this book, this is the one where I can say *"nothing has changed over time"* relating to how I prioritise patient care and delegate to staff today. In contrast to the supernumerary status afforded to student nurses nowadays, however, I experienced the reality of prioritising care before I qualified.

Although student nurses today are used to managing individual cases, many do not consider delegating to other team members until the latter part of their second year and third year, whilst having to simultaneously work on third year assignments and dissertations. In the future, nurse education will evolve, as approved educational institutions (AEIs) and their practice learning partners must adhere to the new NMC (2018) standards of proficiency for registered nurses. New graduate nurses will be required to competently lead and manage nursing care delivery, and demonstrate team working and delegation skills at the point of registration. The newly qualified registrant will also be expected to support and supervise other students and provide constructive feedback on their performance (NMC, 2018).

Newly qualified nurses often have a big learning curve to develop skills relating to team working, time management, prioritising care and delegating to others when they first qualify. Currently, many third year student nurses may care for a lower number of patients than what is expected on registration; for example, four adult inpatients as a third year adult nursing student, in comparison to an average of eight adult inpatients on registration. In the future, third year student nursing competencies should reflect the reality of normal registered nurse caseloads, which will help to prevent the *'reality shock'* that some newly qualified nurses experience when they start in practice. It is better for third years to experience normal caseloads whilst supernumerary and under direct supervision, than when they are a new starter counted in roster numbers.

I have yet to find a third year nursing student who does not find it hard balancing their theoretical work with their practical skill development during their final sign-off year. In line with the new skills-based NMC (2018) standards, universities should review assignment deadlines to allow students time to focus on developing their practical skills. For example, having no assignments or dissertations to complete during final managerial placements would allow third years time to concentrate on consolidating their leadership and managerial skills.

Prioritising care and delegating to team members are skills that are only really acquired through experience. There is a need for employers to actively support newly registered nurses and provide mandatory preceptorship programmes, which includes direct supervision to develop newly qualified nurses' skills in prioritising care and delegating to others. Within my own local NHS foundation trust, a mandatory *'Foundation Preceptorship Programme'* was established in 2015 to support skill development across our trust for all newly qualified nurses (Forde-Johnston, 2017).

My personal view is that every newly qualified nurse should have a mandatory supernumerary period of three months (minimum) when they qualify, and every nurse employer should provide a mandatory national standard of year-long preceptorship. Standard preceptorship would include working alongside experienced nurses for a minimum of 40% of their clinical time during their first 3 months qualified. Currently, there is no national mandatory standard for preceptorship across the UK.

When you qualify, it is important to check the practical supervision and training support offered to develop your managerial and leadership skills during your preceptorship year. You may have band 5 competencies relating to 'team working,' 'prioritising', 'time management' and 'delegation' in practice, that proactively aim to develop these essential skills further when you qualify. Developing skills to prioritise your care and delegate to others is not difficult, but you need to develop these skills through numerous experiences that cannot be learnt overnight. Receiving constructive feedback on your practice from expert role models is an essential part of your future skill development (see the sample preceptorship feedback form in *Box 2.1*).

5.2 HOW TO PRIORITISE YOUR CARE AND MANAGE YOUR TIME

Managing your time and deciding what to prioritise first, when you have numerous call bells ringing, children crying, houses to visit or appointments to get through, can feel overwhelming to any newly qualified nurse (it also feels overwhelming to experienced nurses!). As a nurse, not only do you have to cope with constantly prioritising patients' needs, but you need to be flexible, as humans are not inert beings. Individuals have fluctuating conditions and needs, which you must constantly reassess, to be able to prioritise and respond to when required.

When you qualify, no one expects you to know how to assertively manage all fluctuating clinical situations and individuals' deteriorating conditions. In fact, I am concerned when a newly qualified nurse shows no nerves, is over-confident and asks no questions when they start. Sharing your concerns with experienced staff allows skilled nurses to support you and helps ensure you are providing a safe standard of care.

Start by prioritising your own support and talk to your team

I have never met a colleague who has not felt overwhelmed at some point during their working week, as they could have made a better decision when prioritising or delegating care. Experienced nurses, including myself, will still have odd *'bad days'* where the outcome of a decision does not go to plan. Competent experienced nurses understand the importance of prioritising their support during challenging times and using a team approach. They will talk to each other for reassurance and to debrief or *'let off steam'*. Otherwise, they are at risk of burnout and stress-related illness (see *Chapter 9*).

My top tip, to help you prioritise, manage your time and delegate care to others, is to firstly:

"Prioritise your support!"

Prioritising your support includes three key areas:

1. **Prioritise your needs**
2. **Ask for help and talk to your team**
3. **Reflect and receive feedback from experienced nurses**

If you maintain these three elements during your first year qualified, you will have a supportive foundation to develop your managerial and leadership skills as a band 5. Below are shown some strategies to guide your skill development in relation to prioritising care, managing your time and delegating in practice, using these three pointers.

Prioritise your needs

- **Keep everything in perspective**: it's easy to *'beat yourself up'* and be overly critical, as you want to do your best. Don't be hard on yourself if you struggle to delegate and manage your time. You are not the only new nurse to struggle with documentation at the end of your shift.

- **Don't take work home with you**: life is too short to be regularly worrying about what you forgot to manage or delegate at work. Try to *'switch off', as* everyone has times when they could have performed better. Talking about your concerns with other team members will prevent you worrying at home.

- **Look after yourself physically and emotionally**: it is important for you to *'switch off'* and enjoy your days off. However, regularly staying out late and abusing your body through unhealthy habits is draining. If you are not *'good to yourself'*, and don't make time to relax, keep fit, or eat/sleep well, you are more likely to burn out and make bad decisions. Take time off if you feel excessively physically/emotionally drained.

- **Share practice experiences**: share experiences with other new starters to place them in context. Keep in touch with students you trained with and talk to experienced colleagues. Attend any band 5 supervision sessions offered or access employer assistance schemes.

- **Take breaks**: if a nurse in charge tells you to go for break, then go. Tired nurses make poor decisions and using a team approach means other staff should cover your patient caseload.

Ask for help and talk to your team

- **Ask for help**: when struggling with care, never hesitate to talk to your team and ask colleagues for help. If you are on a ward always pair up with other nurses for support. Don't be afraid to bleep/telephone senior staff for additional support from other team members, as they are there to support you.

- **Access education**: talk to senior nurses/educators about available training to help you, e.g. assertiveness training. Book meetings with senior nurses well in advance (email may be easier). Utilise educational support offered, e.g. is there structured practice supervision, a band competency framework or local preceptorship programme?

- **Find out about your team**: talk to senior nurses and the team about the different roles within your area, how the team works, when they meet together and how your skills can benefit the team.

Reflect and receive feedback from experienced nurses

- **Use a reflective diary**: identify areas where you require assistance and write reflections that focus on your 'time management', 'prioritisation', 'delegation' and 'team working' to share with others.
- **Use practice supervision**: ask for feedback on your practice from experienced nurses to develop your future skills prioritising and delegating (see practice feedback form in *Box 2.1*).

How to prioritise patients' needs and manage an allocated caseload of patients

Some newly qualified nurses are better at prioritising and managing their time in practice than others, be it through their life experiences or having innate leadership skills. Remember that managerial and leadership skills can **always be learnt** and improved through observing good role models and receiving constructive supervision and feedback.

Whilst working with various staff over the years, I have noticed that those individuals who struggle with managing their time tend to do one or all of the following:

- Focus on prioritising one patient (or task) at a time, without enough consideration of the whole caseload
- Focus on perfection whilst carrying out one task, to the detriment of the other tasks required
- Fail to communicate with other team members or ask for help as they see it as a sign of weakness, are too under-confident or have a poor/weak team leader
- Fail to offer to help others, as they are overwhelmed with their own workloads or lack support from their team
- Fail to see the global view or other people's perspectives/workloads
- Have additional concerns/stresses in their life (see *Table 9.5* for more information on band 5 support).

The reality of working in today's NHS means that you cannot aim for perfection all the time; it is not realistic or feasible amid increased vacancy rates and waiting lists. You have to learn to compromise, delegate and prioritise, whilst ensuring that your care is empathetic, patient-focused and safe.

There are four key strategies that newly qualified nurses can use to help them identify patients' priorities and manage an allocated caseload of patients. Firstly, they need to identify immediate patient needs and priorities. Next, they must establish 'urgent/non-urgent' and 'essential/non-essential' nursing priorities and key tasks across their caseload. They then should order or rate these key priorities and tasks, and learn to manage their time efficiently. There are many ways in which these strategies can help you prioritise patients' needs and manage an allocated caseload:

Identify immediate patient needs and priorities

- **Handover data**: understand patients' immediate needs through patient handover/caseload reviews and care plans. Review patients' medical, nursing and MDT notes. Never be afraid to ask questions in handovers if you are unsure of certain terms being used or details being handed over.

- **Introductions**: immediately after a ward handover, always visit each patient you are allocated, to introduce yourself and inform them when you are going home so they know who is taking over from you. Make a mental note of what the person looks like (this is helpful to know if they try to abscond later). During introductions obtain observational/verbal information to help you prioritise care. If you meet an individual for the first time in the community use the same strategies. Experienced nurses continuously assess and reassess patients' needs, during simple introductions and conversations. The data obtained during these encounters allows you to prioritise care at the start of your shift/home visit/clinic appointment. If you feel something is *'not quite right'* with the patient, but are not sure what it is, never hesitate to ask a senior nurse to assess them too, as this is what we are there for.

- **Understand individuals' preferences**: through open questioning, you can establish how individuals feel and what *'they'* perceive to be *'their'* priorities/goals. For example, ask *"How do you feel?"*, *"Are you happy with your care so far?"*, *"Do you have any questions about your care?"* and *"How can I help you?"*.

- **ABCDE approach**: during patient assessments, always use a systematic ABCDE approach to prioritise immediate critical care for adults or children:

    A – Airway: is their airway sufficient?

    B – Breathing: is their breathing sufficient?

C – Circulation: is their circulation sufficient?

D – Disability: what is their level of consciousness?

E – Exposure: anything else to explain the patient's condition? (Resuscitation Council UK, 2015)

Get in the habit of using ABCDE for all patient assessments even when they are stable and 'non-acute'. An ABCDE approach enables you to establish a baseline on which to assess any future deterioration.

- **Prioritise immediate risks to the safety of the patient or others:**
  - Is the patient displaying signs of self-harm, severe depression / anxiety, psychosis, or suicidal thoughts?
  - Is the patient immediately at risk, e.g. choking, haemorrhaging, electrocution or falling at home?
  - Are there risks to other individuals or staff in the vicinity, e.g. severe signs of abuse or aggression / violence?

Establish 'urgent / non-urgent' and 'essential / non-essential' nursing priorities and key tasks across the caseload

- **Distinguish between '*urgent / non-urgent*' and '*essential / non-essential*' priorities and tasks:**
  - an urgent priority will always be '*essential*': urgent or life-threatening priorities are identified through an ABCDE approach and assessment of immediate risks to patient safety. Urgent priorities should be managed and dealt with immediately, through escalation and appropriate team interventions (see *Chapter 8*).
  - a non-urgent priority that is '*essential*': a dressing that needs to be changed that day, or a patient wanting to speak to the doctor about their operation tomorrow are '*non-urgent*' priorities but '*essential*'. They are '*essential*', as a dressing that is not changed can lead to an infected wound and all patients have a legal right to an informed consent. It is '*essential*' you prioritise these tasks that day; however, they are not time-specific. Although, if a patient wanted their spouse present when a doctor spoke to them about life-threatening surgery a time parameter would need to be set. Usually, you can spread these tasks over your shift or potentially delegate to the next nurse on shift.
  - a non-urgent priority that is '*non-essential*': taking an individual in a wheelchair to the shops to buy a newspaper may make them

happy, but is *'non-urgent'* and *'non-essential'*. Taking them to the shops, however, may contribute to holistic care and boost the patient's mood.

- Note: a *'non-essential'* priority may move to an *'essential'* priority, as building a positive therapeutic relationship with a patient, through visiting shops, may lead them to trust you. The trust developed may lead to an individual eventually taking prescribed medication for their mental health that they were previously refusing. Priorities can change and a shop visit could be classed as an *'essential'* priority later for someone with severe depression. When prioritising care across your caseload you must always use an individualised, holistic approach and continuously reassess patients' needs, as they may change over time.

- a long-term non-urgent but *'essential'* priority: a pre-op assessment required for surgery in a month, or a home visit to check an individual can safely climb stairs, are long-term *'essential'* priorities over week or months. Long-term priorities should be documented in patients' care plans, to help future nurses prioritise goals to achieve within realistic timescales (see *Section 6.4* for more on how to write individualised patient care plans).

Order or rate the key priorities and tasks across the caseload

- Identify a method to order nursing priorities / tasks: whether you have a number of *'urgent'* or *'non-urgent'* priorities / tasks, it is helpful to rate them in order. You may write key jobs down on paper or use a technical device to hold this data. Establish what works best for you by trying out different methods. Observe how experienced nurses order or rate their priorities and tasks across their caseloads.

- I use a mixture of methods to order my key tasks. I list urgent tasks at the start of my shift in order, or draw a simple grid on my handover sheet with *'due times'* and *'ticks'* on completion, such as key medications, observations or dressings. The methods I use are flexible, according to the tasks and time parameters set. During very busy shifts, I will use simple lists or numbers across my handover sheet prioritising the order to complete tasks. Senior nurses need a global view of the ward, which involves additional lists of jobs to complete that day or over the week / month, e.g. organising staffing when nurses are on long-term sick. Some examples of methods to rate/order your workload are presented below:

- Use a simple list in order of priority (*example from a fictitious morning shift*):

  1. Insulin pump 9am – Mr Jones

  2. Diazepam 9am – Mrs Smith

  3. Pre-med 10am – Mrs Patel

  4. Bed bath and daily redress foot ulcer – Mr Jones

     (Note: no time is set for the bed bath, as I plan to complete the bath in the morning after other tasks. I also show good time management as **two activities are grouped together.** This dressing comes off during the bed bath and will be dressed soon after.)

- Use a **tick box approach** (example from a fictitious handover sheet below):

Name	Diagnosis	Observations	Meds	Bath	Other
Mr Jones	54-year-old with unstable diabetes (insulin dependent) and infected foot ulcer. IV antibiotics.	10am ✓ 2pm	9am insulin pump ✓ 12pm meds	Bath	Dressing after bed bath
Mrs Smith	80-year-old with severe anxiety and confusion. Risk of falls and awaiting brain scan results from yesterday.	10am ✓ 2pm	9am diazepam ✓ 2pm meds		Phone husband
Mrs Patel	28-year-old elective admission for spinal surgery today. Pre-op observations and checklist completed.	8am Pre-op checklist ✓	10am pre-med ✓		

Manage your time 'smartly'

Aim to work '*smartly*': the term '*working smartly*' means you work efficiently, not harder. In the context of delivering '*smart*' care to a caseload of patients, aim to complete the **greatest amount of care in the most time-efficient and safe manner.** Pointers to help you achieve *'smarter working'* are presented below:

- **Planning and preparation:** prior to delivering nursing interventions, spend time rigorously preparing your required resources, such as equipment, documentation or support staff. If you start a bed bath with no towels, or escalate a patient's condition to a doctor with no observations, you waste time looking for these items later. You will need to observe and discuss preparatory requirements with experienced nurses in your area. Taking time to prepare adequately will always save you time in the long run.

- **Increase your competence and skills (especially in your weaker areas):** it takes time to develop knowledge and skills that you can practically apply in your first post. To help you work *'smarter'*, it is useful to invest time in targeting areas that can become time-consuming, where your knowledge is lacking. I often suggest to newly qualified nurses that they use some of their supernumerary time to develop knowledge and skills in areas that are important, but occur infrequently in their clinical setting. It is during these infrequent 'potential' situations that challenges can develop, which can cause newly qualified nurses stress. It is easier for you to deal with issues such as 'care of a body after death'; a patient walking off a ward threatening to 'self-discharge'; 'non-compliance' as a patient refuses medication or a parent refuses treatment for their child; or a 'Deprivation of Liberty Safeguards (DoLS) assessment' to establish mental capacity, if you have read local/national legal frameworks beforehand. Discussing key practices with your preceptor and reviewing local/national policies, in areas that are infrequent, but important, is time well spent (see *Section 7.3*). Identify where related paperwork is stored in case you need it in a hurry.

- **Work to time and set time limits:** new starters sometimes find it hard to set time limits to tasks, whilst caring for a caseload of patients. There will always be days where one patient or relative needs extra psychological or physical support, or an escalating situation needs more of your time. To meet the needs of a group of patients you have to learn to manage your time within the framework of your shift hours. Don't try to overthink your timings at this early stage, just be aware that you cannot spend 2 hours on bed-bathing a patient who is stable and expect to complete the care for the rest of your patients and finish your shift on time. You will naturally align your nursing interventions to timings through the experience of managing caseloads. I usually take no longer than 30 minutes for each full bed bath if I have three patients who need help washing, or 15 minutes for a simple dressing. With experience, I know I can competently complete these tasks in those times (on average) with carers' support. Obviously, I use a flexible approach to timings as individual issues can arise that cannot be pre-empted.

- **Group activities together:** where possible, try to cluster planned activities together during one patient encounter, e.g. group interventions together, such as completing one patient's observations and medications; and educating them how to manage their symptoms at home, during one bedside encounter, home visit or clinic appointment. Community/district nurses will decrease travel time by grouping home visits according to geographic locations. Nurses can complete a number of tasks on four patients in a hospital bay, such as observations, or three home visits in the same street in succession. **Never administer more than one patient's medications at a time**, as you must adhere to standards of medicines administration at all times. You must use an individualised approach, as some patients may be too tired to have numerous interventions at one time. Observe how experienced nurses group their activities together in your particular area and ask them for ideas to guide your skill development.

- **Complete nursing documentation as you go along and write concisely:** try to complete your documentation as you go along, as opposed to writing or typing it all up at the end of the shift. It can be hard remembering facts retrospectively and often staff jot notes down anyway as they go along. Jotted notes need to be rewritten or typed up, which means it is more time-efficient to formally document them at the time of an event. I have odd days when this is not feasible, due to dealing with emergencies, but most of the time it is possible. I prefer to write care plan goals and evaluations in the presence of the patient to promote joint goal planning, which means I evaluate and document care at the same time. Keep your documentation concise and factual, as writing subjective description is a waste of time (see *Chapter* 6 for comparative examples of *'poor and good documentation'*).

- **Be positive and know where to find solutions to barriers:** there will always be odd shifts where you have barriers to challenge you. Try to maintain a positive attitude and place your challenges in context – this will enable you to get through any difficulties. Senior nurses will have seen the worst case scenarios during their career and they can help you view your challenges in context. They can provide data to help you overcome issues quickly, e.g. links to documentation, specialist staff and contacts. Remember to ask senior staff for advice, as all barriers can be overcome using a team approach.

- **Team work and delegation:** where appropriate, delegate to others (see *Section 5.3* for further guidance). Using a team approach to care – for example, working in pairs or with buddies – will enable you to overcome the hardest challenges in the most efficient and safe manner.

5.3 HOW TO DELEGATE TO OTHERS

During your nurse training, you will have observed registered nurses delegating to others and reflected on how you delegate to support workers. You will have completed competencies that require you to care for a caseload of patients using delegation, under the supervision of your practice supervisor. However, as a newly qualified registered *'named nurse'* you are now fully accountable for an allocated group of patients, which can feel daunting at first. Delegation in nursing is a complex skill, and most of your *'learning to delegate'* will actually take place when you have to delegate.

As an experienced nurse, I know when to delegate, who to delegate to and how to delegate, through my past clinical experiences that give me a frame of reference to gauge my decisions. Try to remember that many nurses struggle with delegation at first (I know I did) but through practice and feedback from experienced nurses you will soon build up strategies that work for you. I have role-modelled nurses who delegated well, learnt not to role model 'poor delegators', asked for advice from experienced managers and learnt from my mistakes. You will probably go through similar experiences and use similar strategies during your preceptorship year. Only you can decide what methods work best for you and I hope some strategies in this chapter help you.

The importance of finding out about junior roles within your team

During your orientation period, it is essential that you find out about the roles, responsibilities and qualifications of junior staff (band 2–4) within your team, as this information is key before you delegate.

A few tips to help you are presented below:

- Ask your line manager or preceptor for an overview of key junior roles within your area and their related job descriptions.

- Establish which tasks junior staff are competent to complete.

- Establish any limitations applied to each nursing band in your area, e.g. allowed/not allowed to complete TPR, fluid balance, diet charts, blood pressures, admission details, etc.

- Do not presume that all nurses of a certain banding are competent to carry out the same tasks. Band 2–4 nurses often complete extended training and they may be at different stages in their career, e.g. have a variety of qualifications and amounts of experience (see band 2–4 nursing structures detailed in *Section 3.4*).

- Create good relationships with junior staff, as the more they get to know you, the easier it will be to deliver collaborative care using a team approach.

- When you first qualify, make a point of introducing yourself to all junior nurses in your area and let them know you are looking forward to working with them.

- Make an effort to introduce yourself to new ancillary staff too, such as ward cleaners, clerks and secretaries. During busy times it is helpful to have additional support from these individuals, as they may assist with appropriate phone calls, domestic work, administration and documentation.

Remember, junior staff are more likely to '*go the extra mile*' for you during busy times, if you acknowledge them and treat them with respect.

Strategies to delegate

When delegating in practice, you should start by identifying patients' priorities and establishing the timelines for key nursing tasks required (strategies to achieve this are detailed above). Once you have identified and ordered key tasks across your caseload, you should manage your time smartly by delegating jobs to junior staff.

There are two common mnemonics used to help junior nurses delegate; the 5 Rs 'Rights of delegation' (NCSBN, 1997) (see *Table 5.2*) and the 4 Cs 'Communication of initial direction' (Zerwekh *et al.*, 1997) (see *Table 5.3*).

These two mnemonics provide helpful guides to aid your communication when you direct others (Zerwekh *et al.*, 1997) or to establish what is *'right'* during delegation (NCSBN, 1997).

Table 5.2: The 5 Rs: 'Rights of delegation' (adapted from Zerwekh et al.*, 1997)*

The 5 Rs	Guidance
1. **R – Right task**	Establish whether *it is the right task* for a specific team member The *'right task'* must adhere to local and national standards and procedures The *'right task'* must be within the scope of the nurse's practice/job description
2. **R – Right circumstance**	Assess the patient and/or patient group/caseload to ensure the *'right circumstance'* is in place to delegate The *'right circumstance'*, or situation, to delegate includes being able to complete tasks that have predictable results and minimum risks, such as a repetitive task or unchanging procedure, e.g. a bed bath or filling in a fluid chart
3. **R – Right person**	Delegate to the *'right person'* who must have the required skills and qualifications to competently complete the task delegated The *'right person'* should have the ability, and be in the right frame of mind, to complete the task set, e.g. not overloaded with other tasks or overly anxious
4. **R – Right direction**	Provide the *'right direction'* when delegating; this includes a concise account of the task required, the reason for the task and your expectations, e.g. you expect a staff member to complete a hair wash during patient X's shower between 10am and 11am, as she has not had her hair washed that week The *'right direction'* includes the right communication that could be provided with '4 Cs': clear, concise, correct and complete (see the 4 Cs (NCSBN, 1997) in *Table 5.3*)
5. **R – Right supervision**	Provide the *'right supervision'* when you delegate, through assessing and monitoring nursing interventions Always be prepared to intervene and provide the *'right supervision'* to staff or re-delegate, if required

Table 5.3: The 4 Cs: 'Communication during the initial direction part of delegation'
(adapted from NCSBN, 1997)

The 4 Cs	Guidance
1. **C – Concise** Is your direction concise when delegating?	Directions need to be concise and easily understood when delegating Gauge if your direction is simple enough by asking the individual if they understand what you have asked them to do; ask them to immediately repeat your directions back to you
2. **C – Clear** Is it a clear direction?	Keep directions short and uncomplicated Break down priorities into clear and measurable tasks Clearly state the task required and the person responsible for completing the task Do not use too much jargon or complicated language, as it may be misinterpreted or cause confusion
3. **C – Correct** Is it a correct direction?	The delegated task should aim for a positive end result that is appropriate for the situation / patient's needs, i.e. the work delegated should achieve the desired outcome Be aware of your overall end goals when delegating to others Never delegate tasks that involve incorrect practices or do not follow policies and procedures
4. **C – Complete** Is it complete?	Monitor and check that all aspects of delegated tasks / patient care are completed fully Accurately record individual assessments and evaluations relating to care delivered Assist with completion of care as required

Following my work with newly qualified nurses as a lecturer practitioner, I have created a mnemonic called the '7 Ks' to help newly qualified nurses focus on what they need to *'know'* when delegating in practice (see *Table 5.4*). The '7 Ks' mnemonic contains guidance to focus your knowledge base before, during and after delegation.

Table 5.4: *The 7 Ks: What you need to 'know' when delegating in practice as a newly qualified nurse*

The 7 Ks	Guidance
1. **K** – Know the specific needs of the patients	Know patients' immediate, medium- and long-term needs across the allocated caseload, e.g. by: • using patient and caseload nursing handovers, open communication with patients/family/carers • reviewing medical, nursing and MDT notes and patients' care plans (see *Table 5.1* for more details)
2. **K** – Know the priorities of nursing care	Know how to prioritise care across the allocated caseload and establish which tasks are: • urgent or non-urgent • essential or non-essential (see *Table 5.1*)
3. **K** – Know your timelines	Know the timelines required for key nursing tasks across the patient caseload Know the different methods you can use to order or rate priorities and key tasks (see *Table 5.1*).
4. **K** – Know your staff and resources	Know ability, skills and competence of staff before delegating to them Know whether the person is capable of taking on additional tasks, e.g. are they overloaded? Know which resources/equipment you need to perform key tasks
5. **K** – Know how to delegate	Develop your delegation skills by using reflection, senior nurse support and receiving feedback Know which tasks are appropriate to delegate to specific staff in your team; use structured guidance to help you delegate, e.g. the '5 Rs' (Zerwekh *et al.*, 1997) (see *Table 5.2*) and '4 Cs' (NCSBN, 1997) (see *Table 5.3*).
6. **K** – Know what has been completed by others to evaluate care	Know how well tasks have been completed by others, by observing their performance and receiving patient/relative/staff feedback on their care e.g. check anti-emboli stockings are removed during a bed bath and the condition of the patient's skin has been assessed during their wash Know how to evaluate and document care delivered by others, using the patient's care plan, risk assessment tools, national standards and practice guidelines (see *Chapter 7* for guidance on care plans and risk assessments) – remember: you are ultimately accountable for key risk assessments and evaluations of care within the patient's care plan as the *registered nurse*
7. **K** – Know whether you need to provide additional support or re-delegate	Know whether staff need extra support following your delegated tasks by monitoring their progress, observing them complete tasks and discussing how they are coping with their tasks in practice Reassess changing situations and re-delegate or directly support staff as required

The importance of positive team working

During your training you will have become familiar with Belbin's 'Team Roles' (Belbin, 2015) that are used to categorise a person's behavioural strengths and weaknesses in the workplace. You will have been encouraged to complete Belbin's Self-Perception Inventory (Belbin, 2015) to identify your strengths and weaknesses; for example, you may come out as a 'shaper' who thrives on pressure or a 'team worker' who is a good listener and diplomatic. On the other hand, as a 'shaper' you may offend people's feelings more easily, and as a 'team worker,' be indecisive when placed under pressure.

Using Belbin's inventory is fun to do and helpful to increase your self-awareness and recognise the contribution of other staff within a team. However, your skills require practical application to promote positive team working when you start in practice. You need to identify where you fit in the team and how you can contribute to team-building and a positive working environment.

Tips to promote positive team working when you start in practice

Meet team members and understand roles

- Within health care environments there will be larger teams, such as divisional teams or clinical commissioning groups; and smaller teams at local level.
- Senior nurses should introduce you to local team members in an orientation walk-round, team meeting or handover. If not, ask them to introduce you or proactively make introductions yourself. Use your orientation period to find out about junior and senior roles within your team (see the orientation checklist in *Table 2.2*).
- Identify all types of teams in your practice area, their purpose and who the team members are.
- Establish where your role fits within each team and the roles that you/other members play (this includes interdisciplinary teams, corporate and patient/carer groups).
- Establish how team members influence and contribute to team working, e.g. speak to team members and discuss their roles and how they promote positive team working.

- Identify who makes key decisions in the team, e.g. who decides staffing levels, when you can book agency staff or when you can take your annual leave.

- Attend as many team meetings as you can when you start, as it will help you to gain insights into team working and networking.

- Attend team social events too as they are a good way to learn about others and make friends, especially if you have relocated in your first post.

Establish how teams are structured and how they communicate

- Some meetings will be informal, such as discussion groups for band 5s; others will be formal with an agenda and minutes.

- Identify which meetings it is essential you attend and which are optional, e.g. ward meetings are usually optional, whereas a team awayday on your roster will be essential.

- Establish how teams communicate, e.g. during handovers, incident reviews, ward/team/research development meetings.

- Find out how team communication systems work and whether you need further training, e.g. online referral systems, bleeping/alarm systems, community caseload reviews, ward meetings, doctors' rounds, team awaydays and written/typed documentation.

Offer to contribute to team working

- Do not presume that because you are new to an area that you cannot contribute to a team or influence change. I know many newly qualified nurses who managed to influence change in their first post, e.g. integrating their dissertation findings into practice.

- If minutes are available from team meetings, then make sure you read them to gain insights into areas that need developing.

- If you have a passion or interest then share it with your manager and the rest of the team. You may be allocated time to pursue an area of interest as a link nurse or be allocated related study days/post-registration training (see *Section 9.2*).

- Remember, it is important that every team member has a voice and yours is just as important as that of any other staff member.

- Offering to help other team members will help you develop positive relationships and will usually be reciprocated in the future when you require additional support.

Communicate with team members professionally and honestly

- Always communicate with staff/team members in a professional manner, be it face to face, on the phone, or online. Never lose your temper or shout at others in practice, no matter how frustrated you feel.

- Learn to assert yourself and say how you feel professionally and honestly. This can seem daunting until you get to know team members, but it promotes positive team working and safe nursing care (see further tips on being assertive at the end of *Chapter 2*).

- Don't be afraid to ask other team members for support or escalate a team issue to someone senior/a trusted colleague (see how to escalate in *Chapter 8*).

Promote positive team working and deal with conflicts

- It is essential that negative team cultures and conflicts are resolved, otherwise people become resentful and frustrated. If left unresolved, situations can impact standards of care.

- When team communication breaks down it is stressful for everyone involved and may become life-threatening for patients, e.g. an essential medication or home visit could be missed.

- Relatively minor encounters/interactions between team members can escalate into much more if left unresolved, e.g. an abrupt conversation or email being interpreted differently to what was intended.

- A whole team can be affected by just one or two team members not getting on, especially if other members of the team take sides. An issue cannot be resolved until it is highlighted and junior staff may find it hard to be the first person to highlight an issue. If you feel uncomfortable about the way team members are behaving, speak to a trusted experienced staff member or visit your HR department for confidential advice and support. Senior nurses should lead mediation between team members to promote positive team working and resolve team issues.

- Remember if you report an issue to a senior person you should stick to the facts, not what you *think* is happening from the gossip you have heard (for more information on reporting and escalating incidents see *Chapter 8*). A person being reported for bullying/unprofessional behaviour has a *'right of reply'* and may be told what has been said about them. You may be asked to write a formal statement if you have witnessed unprofessionalism and you cannot refuse if part of an investigation.

- Miscommunication can escalate when others gossip and spread mistruths, or information is shared second/third hand. Don't gossip about other people, even if you hear others gossiping. It causes undue stress for the individuals being gossiped about and prevents positive team working.

Learn to adapt to change and be flexible

- Learning to adapt to change and being flexible when working in a team, are essential skills for nurses to develop, enabling them to cope in unpredictable health care environments. These skills take time to develop when you qualify. Access supervision and support from experienced staff and educators if you are finding it hard adapting your plans.

- Some staff become easily focused on their own caseload and may have less thought for other team members, as they may become overwhelmed with workloads or do not understand what is happening around them. A good team leader will inform staff of corporate or local issues that impact on team working, which makes them more likely to embrace change and work together with a sense of team purpose.

- Spending time with senior staff, caseload managers and ward/floor coordinators in practice will increase your insights into their role and help you gain a more global perspective of leadership and management in your area.

- Remember, in life there will always be certain people you would prefer not to socialise with and personalities that will clash with your own. In society you would walk away or not pick up the phone; however, at work you cannot do this as part of a working team. You need to communicate in a mature and professional manner with all team members.

- If you clash with a certain member of staff and feel an atmosphere developing, it is best to talk it through with them and let them know how you feel in a professional and honest manner. It is best to initiate conversations in a quiet room and not in front of an audience. Listen to their perspective – you may not be best buddies but can aim for a professional relationship in the future.

- Mediation can be offered between you and others if you cannot resolve an issue. HR staff or a senior nurse/union representative can help mediate to ensure a positive conclusion.

Team support in the community and a hospital 'buddy' system

When nurses work collaboratively with others, be it in a community or hospital setting, patient care will inevitably be more effective. Good team work requires structured mechanisms to support and enhance team communication that are embedded within working environments.

Nurses working in community settings may undertake home visits or run practice clinics, usually caring for a caseload of patients in one geographic region. It can be rewarding working across a community setting, enabling people to stay in their homes and out of hospital; however, there may be times when staff feel isolated during visits or whilst running clinics. To prevent feelings of vulnerability as a lone worker, most community teams have clear structures in place to ensure newly qualified nurses feel well supported by colleagues. Sometimes visits or clinics are undertaken by two staff when there are challenging situations to deal with, and you can request extra help from a variety of professionals if you feel worried by a complex case.

Community teams and practice teams offer regular contact with other members of the team, as follows:

- Daily/weekly patient or caseload reviews
- Nursing team, MDT and IDT meetings held in local offices, GP practices or other community locations
- Additional ad hoc case reviews and team meetings for complex and challenging cases/situations
- Ongoing expert support and reassurance offered from senior staff via telephone or online
- Personal alarm systems to ensure staff are supported in emergencies
- Lone worker policies and procedures to assure staff safety (check your local policies and procedures during your orientation)
- Personal iPads, 1:1 professional mentoring or coaching and access to online professional support networks.

If your first post is community based, make sure you find out how to access team support and all the services available to you.

Similarly, when working in hospitals or other institutions a team approach is essential. Although you should have easier access to a team within the vicinity of your workplace, not all teams work cohesively and effectively. The one method I have used throughout my career to effectively manage my time when caring for a group of ward patients, is to 'pair' or 'buddy' all ward staff at the start of my shift.

When you qualify, you will struggle in a ward or theatre setting if you do not have someone to pair up with during your shift. Some nursing interventions require more than one nurse, and having a shift buddy will help you feel more confident when managing your time and priorities. The buddying method is not just for newly qualified nurses either; it is a method that can be used for all ward and theatre nurses throughout their career. Although buddying sounds simple, it is dependent on the nurse in charge, the workplace culture and you being proactive. Not having an allocated shift buddy as a newly qualified nurse can make your shift busy and stressful.

Buddying usually involves the following:

- Trained nurses and/or health care assistants working together in pairs/threes to support each other; cover breaks and deliver interventions that need more than one nurse
- Identified staff buddying at the start of the shift (after nursing handover), to the end of the shift
- Odd numbers of staff placed in a 'threesome' or given a 'nurse floater' role across the ward/clinic
- Ward managers or other senior nurses buddying with you to cover for a trained nurse who has left the ward/clinic/theatre, e.g. to go to theatre or take a patient to another department
- A buddy nurse (preferably trained) caring for your patients during your break
- Negotiated breaks planned in advance with your buddy
- Intermittent meetings with your buddy during your shift to check on each other, e.g. at the start, in the middle and near the end of the shift
- Negotiating and reviewing key interventions being delivered together during the shift, e.g. *"We have two patients who need repositioning four times this shift and two need help feeding. Shall we meet to reposition*

Mrs X at 2pm and Mrs Y at 3pm, as she was repositioned an hour ago? I will ask HCA Z to feed Mrs X at 5pm and I will feed Mrs Y."

- A more experienced buddy guiding the less experienced nurse.

Remember, as a newly qualified nurse you will struggle with time management and developing your leadership and management skills without support strategies being in place or someone to buddy with. As you become a more experienced nurse, you will be able to offer support strategies or use a buddying system to assist junior nurses with their nursing priorities!

REFERENCES

Belbin, R.M. (2015) *Team Role Theory – Belbin Team Roles.* Available at: www.belbin.com/about/belbin-team-roles/ (last accessed 10 June 2018)

Forde-Johnston, C. (2017) Developing and evaluating a foundation preceptorship programme for newly qualified nurses. *Nursing Standard,* 31: 42–52.

National Council of State Boards of Nursing (1997) *The Five Rights of Delegation.* National Council of State Boards of Nursing. Available at: www.ncsbn.org/fiverights.pdf (last accessed 10 June 2018)

Nursing and Midwifery Council (2018) *Future Nurse: standards of proficiency for registered nurses.* Available at: www.nmc.org.uk/globalassets/sitedocuments/education-standards/future-nurse-proficiencies.pdf (last accessed 10 June 2018)

Resuscitation Council UK (2015) *Resuscitation Guidelines 2015.* The Resuscitation Council UK. Available at: www.resus.org.uk/resuscitation-guidelines/introduction/ (last accessed 10 June 2018)

Zerwekh, J., Claborn, J.C. and Miller, C.J. (1997) *Concepts of Nursing. Basic Care Memory Notebook of Nursing.* Dallas: Nurse Education Council.

WHAT TO DO NEXT

1. Establish what practical supervision and support will be offered when you start, to develop your managerial and leadership skills during your preceptorship year, e.g. you may have band 5 competencies relating to *'prioritising'*, *'time management'*, *'delegation'* and *'team working.'*

2. Reflect and receive feedback on your skills from experienced nurses when you prioritise, manage your time and delegate in practice.

3. Review the roles, responsibilities and qualifications of junior staff (bands 2–4) in your area. Establish which tasks junior staff are competent to complete, and the limitations applied to each nursing band. Ask your line manager or preceptor for an overview of key junior roles within your area and related job descriptions.

4. Identify the types of teams in your area, their purpose and communication systems; and how they relate to your role.

5. Find a strategy to help you work positively within your team, prioritise care, manage your time and delegate to others in practice, that works best for you. If you are unsure what to use currently, review the strategies presented within this chapter to help you identify patients' priorities and manage a 'caseload' of patients.

CHAPTER 6

UNDERSTANDING DOCUMENTATION, CARE PLANNING AND CLINICAL RISK ASSESSMENT TOOLS

❝ *Our clients have mental health issues, and it is better to write up nurse–client conversations as you go along, so you don't forget what was discussed.... For example, if clients refuse to take their medications at home, you go through the risks with them to help them to understand how this will affect their mental health. You need to write up facts, stating what has been said by you and the client; for example, "Mr X stated that ..." and "I stated the risks were ...". This has been the biggest learning curve for me. When I first started, my team leader used to check my written notes to improve my style of writing. I used too much description and put what I 'thought' rather than the facts.* **❞**

1 year post-qualified mental health nurse

❝ *I really needed lots of help to write my care plans from scratch when I qualified. I only used standardised care plans as a student or care plans written by mentors. Standardised care plans are great to let you know what you have to do to keep your patients safe.... They're good for post-op care to let you know what observations to do. In my rehab unit we don't just use standardised care plans and I found writing care plans on my own hard at first. The rehab goals on patients' care plans in our unit are always written with the patient, as not every person has the same rehab goals. Goal planning with our patients means I can give true person-centred care and I find them easy to write now.* **❞**

14 months post-qualified adult nurse

When starting in practice, newly qualified nurses may worry about their documentation, such as their responsibility to provide accurate narrative and complete their records before the end of a busy shift. One of the key questions I am asked by newly qualified nurses is: *"How can I improve my documentation and care planning?"* This chapter offers practical tips to help improve your documentation. I have included a section on risk assessment tools, which are a fundamental part of nurses' record-keeping today, to prevent the risk of harm to patients.

6.1 PAST NURSING DOCUMENTATION AND RECORD-KEEPING TODAY

When I qualified as a nurse in the 1980s, nursing documentation and record-keeping was simpler and more basic than today. There was less documentation required; for example, one risk assessment on every patient admitted to our ward to prevent pressure ulcers. Nowadays, nurses have to complete numerous risk assessments using a variety of tools – for example, pressure ulcers, falls, malnutrition, unsafe self-medication, pain, depression, suicide, self-injury and venous thromboembolism (VTE).

Computers were only widely introduced in the health service around the mid-1990s; prior to this, nursing documentation and records were paper-based and there were no email exchanges or electronic alerts between staff and employers. All my post-qualification mandatory training was classroom-based, and communication across health care teams entailed face-to-face conversations, written material or telephone calls. In comparison, there is widespread use of information technology today, such as email, e-learning, electronic health records (EHR) and electronic patient records (EPR). Many areas have begun to use electronic 'point of care' (POC) documentation using medical devices.

Over the years, we have seen an increase in the use of essential documentation, such as mandatory risk assessments and standardised, pre-written care plans. We have higher levels of criticism, complaint and litigation across health care services than in the past. The increase in nursing documentation reflects perceived falling standards across UK health care services and the need to assure the delivery of safe care. Additional records may assure managers that essential nursing interventions have been carried out safely and the risk of individual harm decreased, but only if documentation is completed accurately and on time.

6.2 THE IMPORTANCE OF DOCUMENTATION AND RECORD-KEEPING

Nursing documentation and record-keeping has two key functions; firstly, to **communicate relevant clinical information**. Examples of the documentation and forms used for this include:

- nursing handover and patient transfer forms
- admission and discharge forms
- ward round notes
- care plans – assessment, planning, implementation and evaluation of care
- patient care pathways
- multidisciplinary plans
- observation charts
- medication administration charts
- fluid balance and diet charts
- case conference and multidisciplinary meeting notes
- ward meeting agendas and minutes
- patient/relative communication diaries.

The second function of nursing documentation and record-keeping is to **support adherence to national and professional standards, policies and law** relating to prescribed care. Documents used to this aim include:

- checklists for assurance, e.g. turning charts/intentional rounds, hourly drainage/pump charts
- escalation and early warning charts
- storing valuables form
- risk assessment tools
- Deprivation of Liberty Safeguards (DoLS)
- mental capacity assessment forms
- restraint forms
- Do not Resuscitate (DNR) or withdrawal of treatment forms
- sectioning forms

- pre-op checklists and consent forms
- self-discharge forms
- death certificates
- incident reports
- audits
- non-adherence, omissions and refusal of care forms.

A *'good'* standard of record-keeping and nursing documentation is essential (see *Box 6.1* for a summary of reasons why you should maintain good standards).

Box 6.1 Reasons to maintain good standards of documentation and record-keeping

- To provide effective communication between health care professionals.
- To maintain continuity of care plans and delivery of safe, evidence-based care.
- To provide important time-lined data to investigate complaints or incidents.
- To assure care to prevent future complaints and legal claims (there is an increasing willingness to 'sue' following an increase in law firms encouraging personal injury claims and media attention on cases of malpractice).
- To provide evidence during inspections and audits (may be national CQC inspections or local audits).

Professional standards and competence

As a newly qualified nurse, you will already be aware of the NMC (2015) *Code of Professional Standards of Practice and Behaviour for Nurses and Midwives*. The need for accurate record-keeping, according to this Code, is drummed into you from your first year of nurse training. You will have passed a documentation competency under the supervision of your practice supervisor to show adherence to the NMC (2015) professional standards, such as:

- keeping *'clear and accurate records relevant to your practice'*
- recording documentation *'at the time or as soon as possible after an event'*, to ensure your colleagues have *'all the information they need'*
- recording *'clearly written'* documentation that is *'dated and timed'* with no needless *'abbreviations, jargon or speculation'*

- keeping your records secure at all times to maintain patients' confidentiality.

New NMC (2018) standards of proficiency call for registered nurses to clearly demonstrate the *'ability to keep complete, clear, accurate and timely records'* and to *'work in partnership with people to develop person-centred care plans'*. On qualification, your understanding of key national and local documentation standards will be of a *'competent'* level; however, you may find it useful to review your nursing documentation standards and writing style, especially when writing care plans. Some examples of *'poor'* versus *'good'* nursing documentation are presented later in this chapter to guide you further.

The implications of poor documentation

As a registered nurse, you have a professional and legal duty to provide clear and accurate documentation and records. A common reason for NMC misconduct cases includes the *'significant failure to keep proper records'* (NMC, 2016). The implications of poor documentation and record-keeping can be devastating for patients and relatives, and your career. All of the disciplinary and performance and conduct cases I have been involved with during my 30-year career have involved poor or missing nursing documentation *(thankfully, such cases are very rare!)*. The potential implications of unclear, inaccurate or missing documentation are summarised in *Table 6.1*.

6.3 THE DIFFERENCE BETWEEN 'GOOD' AND 'POOR' DOCUMENTATION

The above heading presents a choice between *'good'* or *'poor'* documentation, which belies the fact that some newly qualified nurses may feel their documentation is somewhere between the two ranges. As a newly qualified nurse, you should already know the importance of presenting an accurate account within your documentation that is non-offensive and does not breach patient confidentiality. You may benefit from reviewing practical examples of documentation to develop your documentation skills further.

When supporting newly qualified nurses to develop their documentation and record-keeping in practice, I cover the following three key areas: **legible and clear handwriting/typed narrative; correct, actual and professional meaning; and a concise and factual writing style.**

Table 6.1: The potential implications of poor nursing documentation and record-keeping

The effects of unclear, inaccurate or missing documentation	Examples of implications in practice
Ineffective communication between health care professionals	Vital information missed that can cause harm Increased risk of poor care, that is unsafe and substandard, can lead to: • increased readmission rates due to unsafe discharge and post-discharge complications • extended stay in hospital • complications due to poor, incorrect or missing care • failed care packages in the community and increased readmission rates • incorrect drug administration leading to omissions and drug errors • incorrect nursing interventions being administered • increased risk of deteriorating patients due to lack of documented observations
Lack of continuity of care plans and safe, evidence-based care	Incorrect care and omissions, leading to poor patient outcomes and complications (as above) Increased risk of safe nursing indicators, e.g. falls, pressure ulcers, depression, suicide, dehydration and malnutrition, due to lack of documented risk assessments Risk of operations, treatments, interventions and investigations being cancelled Risk of malfunctioning equipment pump causing overdose Increased risk of injury / patient deterioration / death due to lack of escalation
Lack of assurance from timelined data to investigate complaints and incidents, or deal with legal claims	Lack of evidence to answer a patient / relative complaint, internal investigation or external legal claim *(remember, if it's not written down, it didn't happen in the eyes of a court, and narrative will assist your defence)* Increased risk of being personally sued and liable for a compensation claim
Lack of evidence during inspections and audits	Increased risk of disciplinary procedures due to a lack of adherence with local and national standards; professional and legal benchmarks during audits Increased risk of your service being closed by the CQC or local employer / council

Legible and clear handwriting/typed narrative

- If handwritten, use black ballpoint pen (blue pen fades over time); do not use fountain pen as ink smudges.

- Include full date, year and time on documentation (always use 24-hour clock).

- Use clear handwriting, or competently key in text to computer, to enable reader to understand your text.

- Sign all documentation entries (includes electronic) as soon as possible after an event (clearly sign and print your full name and role).

- Never leave lines/gaps between words that can be filled in later.

- Avoid unnecessary jargon, slang or abbreviations, e.g. 'CT' may be short for chemotherapy or computerised tomography (CT scan).

- Never remove entries or use Tippex (always draw a single line through incorrect words and make clear what was originally written and why changed). Check the correct procedure with your employer for errors using computer systems.

Practical comparative examples of documentation relating to legibility of narrative are shown in *Box 6.2*:

Box 6.2 Comparative examples of legible and clear handwriting or typed narrative that adheres to the NMC (2015) Code

Example 1: *"Early shift 4pm, 24ᵗʰ January:*

On-call doctor asks for Jane needs a……… CT in our other unit, but I can't take her as too busy to go. …………She rides on bed now with late nurse at end of list. Name/Role Staff Nurse Late shift and Signature:……………"

Example 2: *"Date: 24.01.2018 at 16.00hrs*

Dr Forde (Senior Registrar on call) has requested that Mrs Smith has a Computerised Tomography (CT) scan of her head today. Nursing staff are waiting for the time from the scanning department receptionist who stated that it will take place at the end of today's scanning list. Please ring the scan room reception on the internal telephone number 123456 if needed. There is no preparation required for Mrs Smith's scan. Dr Forde has explained the reasons for the scan to Mrs Smith and she has consented to the scan taking place. Dr Forde has requested that a nurse bleeps him if Mrs Smith has not had her scan by 17.00. Name/Role: Staff Nurse Sue Hill and Signature: Sue Hill."

Explanation:

Example 1 is ambiguous, unclear and unprofessional. *Example 2* is easy to understand, precise and more legible.

The following key areas within *Example 1* are incorrect:

- A specific date with the year is missing.

- The 24-hour clock is not used; *'4pm'* should be *'16.00'* instead.

- The surname of the patient, doctor and nurse is not given, nor are the role of the nurse and doctor and the nurse's signature.

- Confusing language is used, such as *'on-call doctor asks for Jane needs'.* It is unclear what is meant here; did the doctor ask Jane anything or does she need a scan?

- There is unprofessional use of slang, i.e. the term *'rides on bed'.*

- There is improper use of the abbreviation *'CT'*, in contrast to a full explanation of *'Computerised Tomography'* in *Example 2.*

- The non-specific use of the words *'in our other unit'* could be misinterpreted, whereas full factual details relating to the planned scan are given in *Example 2.*

- There are inappropriate gaps between words that could be filled in retrospectively.

Additional tips:

- Never write *'on-call doctor'.* You must always state the doctor's role and surname, as centralised rotas may change or become lost over time.

- Some areas may use well-known abbreviations such as BP for blood pressure, or a neuroscience ward may regularly use CT of head/spine. Check what is acceptable by your line manager; however, we should generally avoid using abbreviations in practice to prevent confusion.

Correct, accurate and professional meaning

- Written or typed narrative should be clearly understood and not ambiguous or unprofessional.

- Always record accurate documentation that is factually true, e.g. never complete documentation before events happen or falsify text.
- Write precisely using correct documentation, evidence and timelines, e.g. correct observations recorded at right time in the right patient notes.
- Maintain professionalism when writing about a patient, relative or colleague with no insulting, derogatory or inappropriate comments.

Practical comparative examples of documentation relating to accuracy of meaning are shown in *Box 6.3*:

Box 6.3 Comparative examples of correct, accurate and professional meaning

Example 1: *"09.00am I came on my early shift and the agency night nurse was very rude to our morning Nursing Assistant Ruth Rain. I have complained to our Ward Sister about her rudeness to staff and rang up the agency to complain. Otherwise Mr Smith was not in pain this morning and he settled well. His wound did not leak and his urinary catheter is patent, bowels opened 2 times +++. IV continues and IV Venflon tissued this morning. No more fluids planned and no need to re-insert IV Venflon. Patient back from theatre 24 hours ago. Patient vomited and feels nauseous and pain meds given at midday."*

Example 2: *"10.00 Mr Smith stated that he had no back pain and that his pain score was 0. His observations were normal BP 120/80mmHg, Pulse 80bpm, Temp 36.8 degrees C.*

12.00: Following a full bed bath this morning, I observed Mr Smith's post-op wound dressing on his lower back. No oozing, redness or signs of infections noted around his back operation site. Mr Smith has passed 500ml of clear urine since 06.00 with no signs of urine infection.

At 13.00: Mr Smith complained of abdominal discomfort and passed 2 watery bowel movements in succession. A stool sample was taken and sent for culture and sensitivity. Unable to record exact amount of stool passed due to its watery consistency.

At 13.30: Mr Smith vomited 200ml once and 50mg of IM cyclizine given with good effect, with no vomiting witnessed since. Dr Forde (House Officer) contacted and he will resite Mr Smith's IV Venflon at 15.00 if patient is not tolerating fluids by 15.00. At 14.00: Mr Smith stated that his back pain is now scoring 1 and 50mg of IM tramadol given at 14.00 as prescribed."

Explanation:

Example 1 is less specific, inaccurate and more unprofessional than *Example 2*. *Example 2* records accurate timelines of specific events and expected nursing actions and evaluation. The following key areas within *Example 1* are incorrect:

- Unprofessional information is inappropriately shared within the patient's care plan, detailing a dispute between nursing staff.

- Inaccurate timelines are used, 09.00 for the whole narrative, which suggests all the events that morning happened at 09.00. This is obviously inaccurate as the nurse states that medication was given at midday.

- There is a lack of nursing assessment and evaluation shown, e.g. amount of fluid urinated and signs of infection.

- More specific detail is required relating to nursing actions, such as a pain assessment score and the relief of vomiting and nausea.

- There is a lack of assurance that care delivered is of the standard expected. The nurse states Mr Smith does not need his IV Venflon re-inserted when he is at risk of dehydration, due to his lack of IV access and nausea and vomiting 1 day post-op. In contrast, *Example 2* nurse provides assurance that the care provided has been safe. She states her specific actions, such as giving anti-emetics with good effect and the plan for a doctor to re-insert a Venflon at 15.00.

- The nurse in *Example 2* is problem-solving and using the Nursing Process to implement appropriate interventions, such as taking a stool sample for culture and sensitivity (see *Section 6.4* on individualised care planning).

Additional tips:

- Always double-check your narrative for accuracy and read text through before signing.

- If you cannot write events up straight away, make a brief note of times and events on your handover sheet (so you do not forget timelines).

Concise and factual writing style

- Keep sentences short and concise by recording specific facts according to timelines, e.g. what was observed or what was actually said.

- Language used should be clear and simple. Do not over-elaborate language using complicated words or 'flowery' description.

- Only use adjectives if they add context to the situation, e.g. '200ml of urine passed that was a *"rose"* pink colour'.

- Language used should be objective and non-judgemental, as opposed to subjective and emotive. Never document comments about your perceptions or opinions of the person or a family situation. It is a waste of your words and time, and can make you seem judgemental and uncaring.

- When a difficult event occurs you must document it by recording the evidence and facts, as if you were writing a crime report as a police officer who could go to court with that report.

Practical comparative examples of documentation relating to a concise and factual writing style are presented in *Box 6.4.*

Box 6.4 Comparative examples of writing style

Example 1: *"Mr Smith slept well and had a pleasant morning, but his dementia got worse at lunchtime. He made me very upset by being so rude and he was shouting and being very aggressive to staff. I have complained to the nurse in charge about his behaviour in case it happens again this afternoon. Mr Smith is happy and pleasant for 10 minutes then he is really rude again. When he was like a 'mad man' at lunch I left him with our HCA, as he gets on with her better than me. Mr Smith's wife is coming in this afternoon and I can talk to her about his behaviour and what to do with him. She seems relieved when she comes in as we are giving her a break by looking after him in hospital."*

Example 2: *"Mr Smith stated that he did not sleep well when asked by me this morning as he 'heard a baby crying all night'. I reassured him that there was no baby and we could give him his favourite hot milk tonight to see if it would help. Mr Smith slept for most of the morning and when he woke up at 12 midday he was shouting to go home. When I sat with him he swore twice at the door as he thought there were burglars entering, then he threw a bottle of urine at the door. We tried to calm Mr Smith down with music and I asked his wife to speak to him on his mobile, which calmed him down quickly. Our HCA Jenny Jing sat with Mr Smith and read to him; that settled him down and he stated he felt 'happy as no one is in my room now' after his lunch. I have arranged for Mr Smith's wife to meet Dr Forde at 14.00 to discuss his current condition."*

Explanation:

Example 1 is emotive, subjective, uncaring and unprofessional. In comparison, *Example 2* is precise, factual, caring and professional.

Key areas within *Example 1* that are inappropriate include:

- Stating that a patient has had a *'pleasant'* day or *'slept well'* is conjecture and opinion. The only person who can say they *'slept well'* and are *'happy'* is the patient themself. Only write such comments if they are accompanied by "Mr Smith *'stated that'*; *Example 2* nurse writes *'Mr Smith stated that he did not sleep well when asked by me this morning as he heard a baby crying all night'*.

- When a patient displays signs of aggressive behaviour you must document this. However, it should always be written in a factual and professional manner. State what the person *'did'* and *'said'*, as it may indicate a reason for the behaviour. *Example 2* handover has detailed how to calm Mr Smith down, such as reading to him and playing music. The nurse states that Mr Smith has sworn and thrown a bottle of urine, which is factually correct. These facts provide important information to the next shift that will now have an increased awareness that Mr Smith may display signs of anxiety and aggression.

- Unprofessional statements are written in *Example 1*, including a complaint about the patient's behaviour to the nurse in charge and that his wife seems *'relieved'* as they are giving her *'a break'*. These comments are inappropriate opinions and there are no facts presented to back them up; did Mr Smith's wife actually state this? Always write as if the patient, family or a lawyer could be reading your documentation and you will naturally write more factually with evidence to back up your statements. If you are a descriptive writer, practise writing more precisely with your preceptor.

- Descriptive *'flowery'* language has been used such as *'mad man'* and *'really rude'*, which is inappropriate, unprofessional and uncaring. Mr Smith cannot help having dementia and this could be one of your family members, or someone you know, behaving in the same manner. You should always treat people and relatives in this situation with compassion. The nurse in *Example 2* makes no emotive judgements or derogatory comments. She shows a caring approach by offering hot milk, an HCA to read to him and a mobile phone call to his wife.

6.4 INDIVIDUALISED CARE PLANNING

An individual care plan should be used for each patient, from admission to discharge, whilst they require nursing care. A care plan is a written document that is continuously reviewed and adjusted throughout a shift, according to the nursing care delivered and its effectiveness. A care plan should be written, reviewed and evaluated with the patient, where possible. When I first qualified, nurses were expected to assess, plan and evaluate the implemented nursing care with their patient, or appropriate relatives/carers. We were encouraged not to write care plans at desks away from patients, as they were deemed to be patients' care plans, not ours.

As a newly qualified nurse you will already know that nurses provide care following the directions found in individualised care plans. Depending on where you were placed as a student, you may have received a narrow or broad range of experiences using care plans; for example, investigative, outpatient or clinic areas care for a more transient population requiring less care planning. Some care plans are found in folders near the end of patients' beds or on a nursing station. In the community, they may be kept in patients' homes or practice settings. You may have experienced electronically recorded or pre-written standardised care plans or those written by nurses from scratch. Mentors/practice supervisors may have comprehensively taught you how to write in care plans, or you may have had limited exposure to care plan records.

A care plan is an essential legal document and the information it contains must be legible, factually correct and professional. The aim of a nursing care plan is to ensure the following:

- **Patients' needs are met using a holistic approach**
- **Care delivered is safe, evidence-based, correct and continuous**
- **Nursing care delivered or not delivered is recorded**
- **Effectiveness of care is recorded through nursing evaluation.**

Care plans are essentially 'live' working documents that focus on the priorities of care for each person. The key benchmark for judging if a care plan is up to standard is whether the next nurse on shift can carry on where you left off. I remember a particular nursing sister who identified a day every month when all the nurses had to deliver care on the late shift without a verbal handover from the early staff, using only the care plans. I would not recommend this today; however, it taught the staff to write care plans concisely, factually, professionally and regularly enough to ensure clear communication was shared across our team.

The Nursing Process

In the 1950s, Ida Jean Orlando conceived the 'Nursing Process' theory that underpins our care plans and nursing practice today (Orlando, 1961). From its conception, the Nursing Process was devised to be:

- cyclical, dynamic and continuous
- problem-solving and goal-directed
- patient-centred and collaborative
- methodical and systematic
- globally applicable.

The original Nursing Process was devised with the four key stages of assessment, planning, implementation and evaluation (APIE) (Orlando, 1961). Following its worldwide application, a fifth process emerged in the USA that included a 'nursing diagnoses' element, usually between the assessment and implementation stage. In the UK you must have extended training to diagnose as an advanced nurse practitioner or nurse consultant.

Although different practice areas may use various headings, care plans usually comprise four key stages (see *Box 6.5*).

Box 6.5 Key stages of the Nursing Process (adapted from Orlando, 1961)

Assessment

- Individual holistic assessment identifies a person's needs and the priorities of care

Goal planning

- Priorities of nursing care written as goals to meet a person's needs

Implementation plan

- Nursing care, interventions and actions to be implemented with rationale by the nurse

Evaluation

- Continuous evaluation of the effectiveness of the nursing care delivered.

Guidance to help you review and write care plans is shown below for each stage of the process.

Assessment (data collection stage)

- To create care plan goals, and plan interventions, the nurse must assess the patient's needs and identify priorities of care.

- The assessment process starts from admission, or initial interview, when the nurse identifies the patient's physical, psychological, social and spiritual needs.

- Usually an admission form, or case note, is used to record initial assessment data. Some admission forms reflect a nursing model to identify specific needs, such as the Activities of Daily Living model (Roper, Logan and Tierney, 1980).

- A complete assessment must be made in collaboration with the patient, to identify priorities of care using an ABCDE assessment, compassionate communication and a holistic approach (see *Section 5.2*).

- Clinical risk assessment tools must be completed as part of the assessment process (see *Section 6.5*).

- A review of medical/MDT notes is required to obtain vital information regarding the patient's condition to inform goals, e.g. future investigations and treatments.

- Remember: assessment is cyclical and the nurse will continually reassess the patient for ongoing changes.

Planning (goal planning stage)

- The goal planning stage must consider the patient assessment and be negotiated with the patient (or their relatives/carers if indicated) to ensure clear expectations are established.

- The focus of the planning stage is to set goals to meet the patient's needs and improve their outcomes.

- The goals set must be person-centred and should involve a two-way process of communication.

- If you use pre-written, standardised care plans you can still add individual goals in collaboration with the patient, where indicated. A standardised pre-operative care plan may have person-centred additions, as shown in the example in *Box 6.6*.

> **Box 6.6 Including personalised goals in a standardised care plan**
>
> **Assessment:** *Mr Jones is very anxious about his anaesthetic and classical music helps to calm him.*
>
> **Goal:** *for Mr Jones to be administered his anaesthetic safely and without delay at 13.00.*
>
> **Rationale:** *to reduce Mr Jones's anxiety prior to surgery using classical music.*
>
> **Intervention:** *ensure that Mr Jones has access to his classical music 1 hour prior to his anaesthetic as it calms him down. Mr Jones has been using the bedside radio earphones to listen to Classic FM.*

Implementation (formulated interventions that include rationale for care)

- The implementation section of a care plan may have different headings, such as *'nursing interventions'*, *'nursing care needed/required'*, *'nursing actions'* or *'implemented nursing care'*.

- The implementation part details planned nursing interventions/care to achieve the goals set.

- Care plans often have a subdivision *'rationale for care'* within the implementation section.

Evaluation (ongoing evaluation of goals and interventions)

- Care plan evaluation involves making a judgement on what works and what needs to be changed relating to the current care plan goals and nursing care.

- The evaluation section details the effectiveness of the interventions carried out under the framework of the care plan.

- Care plans are 'live' documents that require continuous re-evaluation to adjust goals and nursing actions as required. For example, if a goal is achieved, the interventions are discontinued. New problems and goals may be identified at a later stage and goal planning/the care plan process begins again.

6.5 THE IMPORTANCE OF CLINICAL RISK ASSESSMENT TOOLS

Clinical risk assessment tools are specific assessments used to measure the level of risk in particular situations, which may take the form of checklists, boxes or rating scales. There are many clinical risk assessment tools in practice that are specific to the fields in which they apply, e.g. mental health, paediatrics, midwifery or acute/long-term adult care. As a newly qualified nurse, you will have used a clinical risk assessment tool at some stage during your training, as you are signed off as competent to 'assess risk' and 'manage risk' in practice. However, you may have limited experience of completing risk assessment tools or they may have been completed by your practice supervisor.

It is helpful to ask your preceptor to check you are meeting the required standard when you begin to complete clinical risk assessment tools in practice. It is important that you establish answers to the following questions:

- **Which clinical risk assessment tools are used in my area?** There will be important risk assessment tools that you must complete, dependent on where you work. The risk assessments from these tools will inform your care plans and person-centred goals from admission until discharge.

- **How are risk assessment tools completed?** Risk assessment tools are easy to complete and user-friendly, usually involving a rating scale, checklist, tick box or yes/no answer. However, you should check you are completing them correctly during your supernumerary period with the support of your preceptor.

- **How are risk assessment tools recorded?** Are they recorded on paper or electronically? Who is responsible for filling them in and when must they be completed? People admitted to hospital or a care home, for example, must have a pressure ulcer risk assessment within *six hours* of admission (NICE, 2015).

- **Where are the results of risk assessment tools recorded?** The risk assessment tool used will indicate the level of risk to a person that should be recorded, e.g. on the admission form, care plan or case note documentation.

- **What standard, evidence-based nursing interventions are expected if the person is at risk?** There is usually a national standard of nursing intervention expected, dependent on the risk assessment used. If there is a high risk of pressure ulcers, for example, the nurse is expected to adhere to an evidence base that would expect two-hourly repositioning of an immobile patient as a minimum. Following individual assessments, some patients may require more frequent repositioning, e.g. if they are prescribed steroids or have a vascular/skin disorder.

- Remember, the recording of risk assessment tools is very important, as they demonstrate a nurse has identified a person's level of risk and planned interventions to reduce and prevent future risk. If there is no recorded risk assessment, or care plans of nursing interventions to prevent risk, it is difficult to argue that safe care was provided if your care is later questioned.

Clinical assessment tools to assess a patient's risk of developing a pressure ulcer have been used for many years. Examples of these are the Norton score (Norton *et al.*, 1962), Waterlow score (Waterlow, 1998) and Braden score (Bergstrom *et al.*, 1987) and there are numerous other tools used across the health service (a few examples across key fields are presented in *Table 6.2*).

Table 6.2: Some examples of common clinical risk assessment tools

Clinical assessment tool	Aim of tool
Braden score (Bergstrom *et al.*, 1987)	Predicts pressure sore risk, providing an estimated risk for the development of a pressure sore in adults
Braden Q score (Quigley and Curley, 1996)	Predicts pressure sore risk, providing an estimated risk for the development of a pressure sore in children
Falls Risk Assessment Tool (FRAT) Peninsula Health Falls Prevention Service (1999)	Predicts the likelihood of falls occurring, either in hospital or at home
Edinburgh Postnatal Depression Scale (EPDS) (Cox *et al.*, 1987)	Identifies patients at risk of postnatal depression, predicts the likelihood that a new mother is suffering from a depressive illness and the level of severity
Generalised Anxiety Disorder Questionnaire (or GAD-7) (Spitzer et al., 2006)	A screening tool and severity measure for generalised anxiety disorder (GAD)
Visual Infusion Phlebitis Score (VIPS) (Gallant and Schultz, 2006)	A visual infusion phlebitis scale for determining appropriate discontinuation of peripheral intravenous catheters
Malnutrition Universal Screening Tool (MUST) (BAPEN, 2011)	A five-step screening tool to identify adults who are malnourished, at risk of malnutrition (undernutrition) or obese

REFERENCES

Bergstrom, N., Braden, B.J., Laguzza, A. and Holman, V. (1987) The Braden scale for predicting pressure sore risk. *Nursing Research*, **36**(4): 205–210.

British Association for Parenteral and Enteral Nutrition (2011) *Malnutrition Universal Screening Tool*. Redditch: BAPEN.

Cox, J.L., Holden, J.M. and Segovsky, R. (1987) Edinburgh Postnatal Depression Scale (EPDS). *Journal of Psychiatry*, **150**: 782–786.

Gallant, P. and Schultz, A.A. (2006) Evaluation of a visual infusion phlebitis scale for determining appropriate discontinuation of peripheral intravenous catheters. *Journal of Infusion Nursing*, **29**(6): 338–345.

National Institute for Health and Care Excellence (2015) *Pressure Ulcers Quality statement 1: pressure ulcer risk assessment in hospitals and care homes with nursing*. Guideline (QS89). Available at: www.nice.org.uk/guidance/qs89/chapter/quality-statement-1-pressure-ulcer-risk-assessment-in-hospitals-and-care-homes-with-nursing (last accessed 11 July 2018)

Norton, D., McLaren, R. and Exton-Smith, A.N. (1962) *An Investigation of Geriatric Nursing Problems in Hospital*. (Section 9: Pressure sore investigation). Edinburgh: Churchill Livingstone.

Nursing and Midwifery Council (2015) *The Code: professional standards of practice and behaviour for nurses and midwives*. London: NMC. Available at: www.nmc.org.uk/standards/code/ (last accessed 11 July 2018)

Nursing and Midwifery Council (2016) *Advice and Information for Employers of Nurses and Midwives*. London: NMC. Available at: www.nmc.org.uk/globalassets/sitedocuments/nmc-publications/advice-for-employers.pdf (last accessed 11 July 2018)

Nursing and Midwifery Council (2018) *Future Nurse: standards of proficiency for registered nurses*. Available at: www.nmc.org.uk/globalassets/sitedocuments/education-standards/future-nurse-proficiencies.pdf (last accessed 11 July 2018)

Orlando, I.J. (1961) *The Dynamic Nurse-Patient Relationship: functions, process and principles*. New York: G.P. Putnam's Sons.

Peninsula Health Falls Prevention Service (1999) *The Falls Risk Assessment Tool (FRAT)*. FRAT Pack. Peninsula, VIC, Australia: Peninsula Health Falls Prevention Service.

Quigley, S.M. and Curley, M.A. (1996) Skin integrity in the pediatric population: preventing and managing pressure ulcers. *Journal of the Society of Pediatric Nurses*, 1(1): 7–18.

Roper, N., Logan, W. and Tierney, A.J. (1980) *The Elements of Nursing: a model for nursing based on a model for living*. Edinburgh: Churchill Livingstone.

Spitzer, R.L., Kroenke, K., Williams, J.B. and Löwe, B. (2006) A brief measure for assessing generalized anxiety disorder: the GAD-7. *Archives of Internal Medicine*, 166(10): 1092–1097.

Waterlow, J. (1998) The Waterlow card for the prevention and management of pressure sores: towards a pocket policy. *Care Science and Practice*, 6(1): 8–12.

WHAT TO DO NEXT
---

1. Review practical examples of key documentation used in practice, to develop your documentation skills further.

2. If you are a descriptive writer, practise writing more precisely with your preceptor.

3. Review your documentation and writing style with experienced nurses in practice to ensure it meets the benchmarks required.

4. Establish the required standard when using care plans and practically applying clinical risk assessment tools in your practice area.

CHAPTER 7

ASSESSING MENTAL CAPACITY AND SUPPORTING THOSE DECLINING CARE

❝ We all look after patients who can sometimes refuse care, like washes, medications and IVs. I had a lecture on mental capacity during my training but I hadn't come across anyone needing a mental capacity assessment in placement until I qualified. It is really important to understand about assessing a patient's capacity. The result of an assessment can have a massive impact on how you deliver care to a person. It can make the difference between someone going home, or not. It can impact on family communication too, if the patient has the capacity to decide to go home but their family are not happy about the discharge. We have a trust lead to help us carry out capacity assessments if the team want support with the decision, which really helps. ❞

18 months post-qualified adult nurse caring for the older person

❝ When you have a patient in practice demanding to leave, walking off the ward, refusing medications, you think, what do I do first? I was only a month qualified and my patient was 1 day post op; she was also addicted to heroin. She jumped off the bed and ran off the ward with her IV drip attached. The ward sister was brilliant and ran off the ward with me to make sure she was OK. The patient refused to come back to sign the self-discharge form. We persuaded her to wait a few minutes so I could run back to get the bits to take her IV out. Our ward sister said she had capacity so she had the right to leave, we couldn't stop her, and the ward is not a prison. We went through the post-op risks and documented all our advice. We filled in the incident form, let next of kin know.

> *Documentation is really important as the patient can be at risk*
> *when they leave. You must always cover yourself, writing what*
> *you said and did at the time.* 🗣

1 year post-qualified adult nurse

When I support newly qualified nurses they sometimes worry about what to do when a patient declines care or is not adhering to prescribed interventions. According to medical terminology this is termed as being *'non-compliant'*; the word *'compliance'* meaning an *'action of complying with a wish or command'* (Oxford English Dictionary, 2018). The current nursing view is that the term *'compliance'* should be avoided, as it reflects a patriarchal approach, as the clinician decides which interventions are required and the patient passively conforms. However, you may still find nursing audit evaluations, service improvements and incident reports using the terms *'compliant'* or *'non-compliant'* when disseminating findings; for example, they may state that 50% of staff are currently compliant with e-learning or falls risk assessments in practice.

In comparison, terms such as *'adherence'* or *'non-adherence'*, and *'concordance'* and *'non-concordance'*, are preferred as being more patient-focused and collaborative terms to use nowadays. *'Adherence'* is related to a process where treatment options are discussed between the clinician and patient. The patient has an active role and the option of agreeing to interventions, or not. The term *'concordance'* is a broader concept where open discussion should take place between the clinician and patient until they come to an *'agreement'* and *'harmony'* (Oxford English Dictionary, 2018). The term *'concordance'* implies that patients' and clinicians' views are both respected and that patients should take responsibility for their own health. However, if a patient lacks the capacity to make decisions relating to their care, prescribed interventions may need to be carried out by staff against the patient's wishes; for example, if there is a risk to their life or it is in their *'best interests'*.

All nurses can find it hard encouraging a person to accept interventions that are in their best interests, while not sounding so overbearing that they are construed as coercively pressurising the person. Often new starters are concerned with the legal implications of patients declining care. It can also be difficult for family or significant others when there are opposing views relating to complicated ethical decisions, such as whether or not to implement 'Do Not Resuscitate' (DNR) or 'withdrawal of treatment' orders.

Newly qualified nurses' concerns usually relate to three key questions: *"How do I decide if an individual has the mental capacity to make a specific decision?", "What do I do if a patient declines care or prescribed interventions?"* and *"How do I support a patient to receive care that is in their best interests without being coercive?".* This chapter attempts to answer these questions, offering practical advice that is informed by the Mental Capacity Act (DH, 2005a), Deprivation of Liberty Safeguards (DoLS) (DH, 2005b), advanced decisions (ADs; sometimes known as an advance decision to refuse treatment (ADRT) or a living will) and granting lasting power of attorney (LPA) to another person. The chapter presents simple guidance to help you deal with patients who refuse essential prescribed interventions, as you are legally accountable for any omissions in your nursing care.

When I qualified, the Mental Capacity Act 2005 did not exist. However, health care professionals still had to adhere to informed consent procedures for planned interventions. Difficult ethical decisions were influenced by health care professional–patient (or family) meetings and predominantly medical judgements. Ward rounds and community case conferences were traditionally medically dominated and aimed to resolve ethical dilemmas surrounding individual cases. There were fewer national directives to inform decision-making, in contrast to the mental capacity assessments, Deprivation of Liberty Safeguards (DoLS) and advanced decisions (AD) used today. Current NMC (2018) educational standards of proficiency call for newly registered nurses to clearly demonstrate effective assessment of a person's capacity '*to make decisions about their own care and to give or withhold consent.*'

7.1 THE CASE THAT LED TO CHANGES IN THE LAW

In 1991 one particular case, *F v. West Berkshire Health Authority* (UK House of Lords, 1991), led to fundamental changes in law and the eventual creation of the Mental Capacity Act (2005). The case involved the sterilisation of an adult woman with a learning disability and focused on whether doctors had a legal right to 'sterilise' her without her consent. She was deemed by medics at the time to lack the capacity to make this decision herself. The House of Lords maintained that 'Case F' did lack capacity to make this decision and the operation was deemed to be in her '*best interests*'. Following the ruling in this landmark case, no one could sue the medics later for conducting the operation without F's consent. The Mental Capacity Act (2005) and measures added to the Act in 2007

(DH, 2007), such as 'The Deprivation of Liberty Safeguards' (DoLS), are used today as the legal basis to determine whether or not an individual has the mental capacity to consent to a specific decision.

7.2 SUPPORTING AN INFORMED CHOICE

You have been trained to respect individuals' informed choices and the decisions they make. A person may decline care or potential life-saving medical treatments at any time. When an individual declines prescribed care, it is your role initially to explore the person's reasons for declining, in a supportive, compassionate and balanced manner. Conversations should always take place with the individual first but it may be appropriate to involve family members, or an appropriate nominated person/people, if the adult is assessed as not having the mental capacity to make the decision themselves (DH, 2005a).

Need for a compassionate approach

You should always use a compassionate approach when trying to establish why a person is declining care and deal with any barriers affecting their informed decision-making. Your role is to educate the person about their options to enable them to arrive at a positive resolution (see *Box 7.1*).

Case study using an individualised approach

When I first qualified, I remember caring for an 18-year-old lady diagnosed with epilepsy and learning disabilities as a child. She was admitted for a review of her anti-convulsion medication. During nursing handover, I was told she was refusing her medication and would not eat her lunch, no matter who tried to coax her. The staff were all kind towards her during the morning shift and she was placed in a busy four-bedded bay with very chatty patients. I spoke to her mum on the phone to discuss why she might be refusing essential medication and I was told that *'meltdowns'* would sometimes happen in bright lights and in social situations if there were many people talking. I had never cared for someone with these needs before and I realised that I needed to nurse her in a quieter room, whilst sitting with her to slowly explain the medications. Once I did this she swallowed all her medications and was much happier. I wrote her specific needs in her care plan to ensure other nurses would continue her care according to her individual needs. She eventually told me that she always felt like there were *'lots of bracken and thorns around her'* whenever she heard lots of voices, which enabled me to realise just how anxious she had felt.

Box 7.1 Using a compassionate approach when a patient refuses care

Find out why a person is declining care

- Identify why a person is declining your care and ask relatives and significant others, if appropriate.
- Treat the person kindly and try to see the situation from their perspective.
- Ask open-ended questions and use active listening to understand the situation from the individual's perspective.
- Avoid telling a patient off, or saying that they *'must'* adhere to protocol.
- Avoid forceful language as it can make a person feel out of control and patronised.
- If the person is unnecessarily rude, your language should still remain calm and professional.

Deal with any barriers

- Use holistic assessment to identify any barriers, e.g. do they misunderstand due to a hearing impairment? Are they worried about the impact on their home situation?
- Use alternative strategies to promote communication, e.g. non-verbal communication aids.
- Use positive interventions to facilitate collaborative decision-making that benefits the patient, e.g. place urine bottles within easy reach to help a person remain on prescribed bed rest.
- Ask for specialist support if indicated, e.g. refer to an alcohol service to promote abstention.
- Request additional support if the person is being intimidating, making an unreasonable request or putting others at risk.

Educate the person and discuss alternatives

- Provide enough information for the person to make an informed choice.
- If a patient / relative has more knowledge about their condition than you, learn from them.
- Educate the person / relevant others in a balanced and collaborative manner, explaining the benefits of prescribed care and the potential consequences of declining.
- Sympathetically discuss potential solutions or alternatives in a kind manner.

Learn from others

- Don't take personal umbrage when a patient adheres to a request from another person (it can happen to senior staff too!). Be positive that the person is responding to your colleague. Ask your colleagues what strategies they used to promote positive collaborative decisions and document the methods that work in the patient's care plan to promote continuity of care.

- Some patients, for whatever reason, may not warm to you. Reflecting with a senior nurse and your preceptor will enable you to receive support and become more self-aware to move forward with strategies to deal with this if it occurs again.

Try to find a solution

- Allow the person time to think about their options. The person may need time to absorb information before they are willing to change their mind.

- If a patient continues to decline care, try to find a solution through compromise and negotiation. On rare occasions, a nurse in charge may need to realign your patient allocation due to stress caused by a person declining care.

Communication passports

A communication passport is a person-centred booklet to educate others of the support required for children, young people and adults, who may find it hard to speak up about their own needs. More people are using communication passports today as they positively present an individual and do not just describe a set of disabilities. A communication passport details the person's preferences, unique character and the most effective way to communicate with them. Always check whether a person has a communication passport as it contains invaluable information that will inform an individualised care plan.

Help to facilitate a decision when the person 'has the capacity' to decide

Over the years, I have sometimes found the smallest intervention helps to facilitate a positive decision that is *'perceived'* to be in the person's best interest. I use the term *'perceived'*, as what you perceive to be in the person's best interest may not be what the individual feels is right for them. The person may be aware of the risks to their health and, if they have the mental capacity to consent to or decline care, they are allowed to make an *'unwise decision'* that must be respected.

Individuals can make an 'unwise' decision

Some choices made by individuals with the capacity to decide are clearly unwise and unsafe, such as a person walking out of a hospital a few hours after major surgery. Other decisions are not immediately life-threatening, such as not washing for weeks. Even if a person has the capacity to decide not to wash for weeks, you would still be expected to do your best to change their mind if there was a potential risk to their health.

A case example of an 'unwise' decision

During a community visit to re-dress a patient's chronic leg ulcer, it becomes apparent that the patient has not washed for four weeks; they are starting to smell and are unusually unkempt. Even though the patient has the capacity to decide to not wash, you would still have a professional responsibility to sympathetically find out why the person was neglecting themself as part of your role to promote health. The patient would be at risk of poor healing, or further infection, due to their inadequate hygiene. The subject would need to be approached sensitively as there may be a reason for their lack of hygiene. Do they feel depressed and not feel like washing any more? Are they recently bereaved? Do they have an addiction to drugs, or have they cognitively declined? A tentative holistic approach should be used by gently asking open questions to establish how they are feeling generally. You would aim to find out why they are not washing; however, you should not bombard them with blunt questions, which they may find invasive. Through open questioning, active listening and developing a therapeutic relationship, a skilled nurse will be able to establish whether additional referrals are required.

A case example using negotiation and exploring other options

Sometimes exploring alternatives and negotiating with a person will promote a positive collaborative decision that is in a person's best interest. A patient may not adhere to their three prescribed doses of an important anti-depression medication daily, as they are regularly abusing alcohol and are too inebriated to take their tablets in the evening. They forget to take their last dose of the day and they have a hangover in the morning, which means they consistently miss their morning dose too. In total, they are receiving only a third of their therapeutic dose, which may put them at risk of severe depression. The GP may reduce the number of doses to one large dose at lunchtime to increase the chance of them maintaining a therapeutic level of medication. As long as the single dose prescribed is within safe parameters, according to the British National Formulary, and side-effects are closely monitored, this could potentially be a viable option to promote adherence until their addiction is addressed.

Difficult decisions

Life-changing, ethical or end of life decisions may be less clear-cut for all involved; for example, medics may only give a 50/50 chance of survival following a particular intervention or worsening odds for treatments during end-stage cancer. No one can predict the outcome of any intervention, which can make it harder for an individual to decide whether to agree to or decline a treatment on offer.

We rely on global evidence and some individuals are willing to agree to interventions that offer relatively small chances of improvement. They may hope for a breakthrough in research and that *'eureka'* moment to happen. In contrast, others may decline treatments with higher success rates as they risk decreasing their quality of life. For example, they may not be able to stand the thought of losing their hair following chemotherapy. The role of the nurse is to provide the person with the knowledge to understand the current evidence base and options available to them to facilitate an informed choice. Specialist support from advanced nurse practitioners, specialist nurses and oncology and palliative care teams can also help individuals having to make such life-changing decisions.

Learning from others

Occasionally, individuals will only adhere to prescribed care when their spouse or parent requests them to; or they will only accept care from one particular staff member. If your colleague manages to positively encourage a person to adhere to prescribed care, try to learn from their strategies (see *Box 7.1*).

There will always be individuals who will not change their mind and, no matter what strategies you use, they will not take your advice, however detrimental the lack of intervention is to their health. These situations can become stressful for all involved and you should always seek support from a senior nurse if you experience this.

7.3 THE LAW AND KEY POLICIES

Having mental capacity means you are able to make your own mind up about a particular decision. Mental capacity should always be assumed unless you have a clear reason to think otherwise. A mental capacity assessment will confirm whether a person being deprived of their liberty lacks the capacity to consent to, or decline, the prescribed intervention. You must adhere to a strict legal framework when establishing whether an individual *'has'* or *'does not have'* the mental capacity to make the decision (DH, 2007).

If a patient is assessed as **having the capacity** to decline an intervention, then care **cannot** be given without their consent. To actively coerce a patient, or touch a patient to make them receive care, would disregard their personal autonomy and breach the principles of informed consent. A patient with the capacity to decide has the right to refuse even life-saving treatment, and touching them without consent is considered unlawful (DH, 2007). In contrast, if a patient declines life-saving treatment and they are deemed as **not having the capacity** to refuse, then you must adhere to national laws according to best interest decision-making.

Determining the outcome of a mental capacity assessment is very important to all nurses, as it will influence whether you **actively promote adherence** or are **legally required to obtain adherence** using strategies such as restraint. Following the updated Mental Capacity Act (2007), it is now a criminal offence to *'wilfully neglect someone without capacity'*. This means a nurse may be liable if a patient comes to harm due to their refusal to accept prescribed interventions, e.g. if they refuse to take prescribed anti-convulsion medication that later leads to brain damage from uncontrolled seizures.

Mental capacity is only relevant to the decision that needs to be made at the time. Just because a person does not have the capacity to make a decision to leave a nursing home, it does not mean they cannot decide to refuse a bath and choose a shower.

The Mental Capacity Act

The Mental Capacity Act (DH, 2005a) is an Act of Parliament applied in England and Wales that sets out to provide legal protection for vulnerable people who do not have the capacity to make a decision about their own care, due to cognitive brain or mental health disorders. The Adults with Incapacity (Scotland) Act (Scottish Parliament, 2000) is the equivalent legislation in Scotland; in Northern Ireland it is the Mental Capacity Act (Northern Ireland) (Northern Ireland Assembly, 2016). The revised Mental Health Act 2007 (DH, 2007) allows restraint to be used on a person aged 18 years or above, in specific situations only. The Mental Health Act (2007) applies to children who are 16 years and over. Parents cannot override their decision, as they are presumed to be *'competent to give consent'* at this age.

If a child is under 16 the Act will not apply, and the child is assessed as to whether they have enough understanding about the risks and benefits of treatment; this is termed *'Gillick competent'*. Children under 16 who are not *'Gillick competent'* must have parents/those with parental responsibility to make the decision on their behalf.

Deprivation of Liberty Safeguards (DoLS)

Hospitals and care homes must follow a standard process before they deprive anyone of their liberty. Depriving a person of their liberty is a serious matter and restraint should only be used as a last resort if it is in their best interests (DH, 2007). DoLS (DH, 2007) were created to ensure that a decision to deprive someone of their liberty is made according to a strict process and through an appointed authority. DoLS can only be used if a person is being deprived in a **hospital setting or care home**. In other settings the Court of Protection needs to authorise restrictions.

Prior to making a DoLS referral, you **must complete a mental capacity assessment** to be sure the person does not have the capacity to make the decision. If a person is assessed as not having capacity and you need to frequently use sedation or physical restraint to control their behaviour, or if the person needs to be confined to a particular area, then a formal DoLS authorisation must be sought. Prior to making a formal DoLS application you must make every effort to use and evaluate **less restrictive ways** to care.

Authorising a DoLS

DoLS authorisation has two elements: an **urgent** and **standard** authorisation. An **urgent DoLS** application must be completed if there is an immediate need to restrain or restrict a person. A *'managing authority'*, such as a trust, may grant an urgent request if a deprivation of liberty is required immediately. An **urgent DoLS** request usually lasts for 7 days and it can only be applied for once, and extended for 7 days. A **standard DoLS** must be sought for any prolonged period and will not be authorised for longer than 12 months at a time. Authorisation should be revised if circumstances change, as the person may not be deprived of their liberty any more.

A **standard** DoLS must be requested using the correct procedure and documentation that is sent to a *'supervisory body'*, usually your local trust or council (see *Boxes 7.2* and *7.3*).

Box 7.2 Pointers to guide a DoLS application

- Six forms may need completing, depending on circumstances. Forms reflect: past history; the purpose of the authorisation; social situation; details of the mental capacity assessment; any advance decision; and the person's physical, neurological and mental condition.

- Check DoLS policy with your employer and establish where the forms are stored, how to fill them in and where they must be sent. Ask an experienced nurse to check your forms the first time you complete them.

- Once forms are sent, your supervisory office will commission a series of *'best interest'* and *'medical'* assessments to grant or refuse authorisation for deprivation of liberty.

- All assessments must be carried out by trained health or social care professionals *(assessments should not be carried out by someone involved in the person's care)*.

- A minimum of two assessors is required; one must be a doctor with expertise in mental health and the other can be any experienced health or social care professional.

- The maximum length of time for a standard authorisation is 12 months.

- When a standard DoLS is authorised, someone must be legally appointed to represent the person, called a *'relevant person's representative'*, e.g. family member / significant other.

- Family / relevant others have the right to challenge a DoLS through the Court of Protection.

- Before a standard DoLS is authorised, key assessments must always take place (see *Table 7.1*).

***Box 7.3* Assessments required for standard DoLS**

- The person is subject to continuous control or supervision.
- The person is not free to leave.
- The person is over 18 years of age.
- The person is suffering from a mental disorder.
- The person lacks the capacity to decide for themselves about the restrictions that are proposed.
- The proposed restrictions are in the person's best interests.
- Should the person be considered for detention under the Mental Health Act (2007) instead?
- Is there a valid advance decision to refuse treatment that would overrule a DoLS?

Use of restraint

Only **proportionate** restrictions and restraint are advocated by the Mental Health Act (2007) for a person who does not have the capacity to make the decision.

Restraint may include:

- door locks/security systems to prevent an 'at risk' person from leaving an area
- manual restraint, sometimes called *'holding'*, to prevent a person leaving
- medication to calm a distressed person (*must be prescribed within legal parameters*)
- physically removing objects to prevent a person from harming themselves; this may include a drip stand or urinary catheter when a person is attempting to pull them out, or keeping sharp implements away from a person wishing to harm themselves
- manual restraint to administer a prescribed intervention, e.g. inserting a nasogastric tube
- always being in the presence of another person for their own safety, sometimes called 1:1 nursing or *'specialing'*
- isolating a person from others in a confined space for their own safety.

You must **avoid** any inappropriate use of restraint and report any abuse that you witness, such as:

- excessive physical or mechanical restraint, when not required
- verbally demeaning a person
- manipulating a person to make them do what you want
- deliberately provoking and winding a person up
- bullying behaviours.

Restraint can feel frightening and humiliating for the person being restrained and you must always treat them with compassion and professionalism. Following the government response to the Winterbourne hospital abuse scandal in 2012 (DH, 2012), the Department of Health published the policy document *Positive and Proactive Care: reducing the need for restrictive interventions* (DH, 2014), which contains a framework to prevent abuse through restraint. The report advocates minimising the amount of restraint used, only using restraint in extreme circumstances and **eliminating the dangerous practice of face-down restraint.** Staff should always **avoid**:

- physically restraining or holding a person face down on a floor
- physically restraining or holding a person in any way that makes it difficult for them to breathe or affects their circulation of blood
- pressing on a person's ribcage, neck or abdomen or covering their eyes, ears, nose or mouth, as it can compromise breathing.

When you start in practice, find out if restraint is regularly used and the rationale for its use. All employers should adhere to safe practices that are underpinned by national laws. If you feel uncomfortable with any restraint practices that you witness, do not hesitate to escalate and contact higher authorities who can advise (see *Chapter 8*). This may also include community settings where relatives may be restraining a person unnecessarily.

Employers should provide **specialist restraint training** for nurses who need to use physical restraint as part of their role, to ensure they use safe practices. When using physical or chemical restraint, it is important that you always keep up to date with changes to national and professional standards.

7.4 ASSESSING MENTAL CAPACITY

Although mental capacity assessment is used frequently in certain settings, such as care of the elderly and mental health (see *Table 7.1*), all nurses have a duty to understand how the Mental Capacity Act (2005) and Mental Health Act (2007) apply in practice.

Assessment is 'decision-specific' and 'time-specific'

A mental capacity assessment is *'time-specific'* and will only apply at a specific time for a specific circumstance. Every case is individually assessed and a person's capacity must be *'decision-specific'*, meaning every decision requires a separate assessment. Just because a patient does not have the capacity to sign their will, immediately post-stroke, it does not mean they cannot decide to have a bath instead of a shower. If there is cognitive improvement months later, they may be deemed as having the capacity to sign their will in the future.

Table 7.1: Conditions that 'may' impact on the capacity to consent

Condition	How it may impact
Dementia	Individual with dementia **may** suffer from memory loss, be forgetful and unable to retain or understand information
Learning disability	Learning disability **may** affect a person's understanding and cause them difficulty understanding complex information, or coping with making decisions
Head or brain injury, or stroke	Severe head injury, brain injury or stroke **may** cause short-/long-term neurological impairment and deterioration in conscious level, affecting the ability to retain information and understand language
Mental health condition	A severe mental health condition **may** lead to altered perspective, hallucinations or delusional thoughts that cause a temporary loss of capability to make decisions for a period
Metabolic disorder	A metabolic disorder, such as diabetes, **may** lead to deterioration in consciousness level or cognition
Poisoned or excessive alcohol/drugs	Similar to a metabolic change, this category also includes post-anaesthetic, which can decrease conscious level

How to test mental capacity

You must always clarify the decision that the individual needs to consent to, and adhere to the five principles of a mental capacity assessment (see *Box 7.4*). When deciding whether an individual has the capacity to make the decision or not, a two-stage mental capacity test must take place (see *Box 7.5*).

Box 7.4 The five principles of mental capacity assessment (DH, 2007)

1. Mental capacity is presumed unless it is demonstrated that the individual lacks capacity.

2. Individuals must be supported to make their own decision and all practical steps must be taken to help them to do so.

3. Just because a person makes an *'unwise'* decision, it does not mean they lack capacity.

4. An act or decision made for or on behalf of an individual who lacks capacity must be made in that individual's *'best interests'*.

5. The *'least restrictive options'* to the individual's *'rights and freedom of action'* should be chosen.

Box 7.5 Summary of the two-stage mental capacity test (DH, 2007)

Stage 1: Is there an impairment or disturbance in the functioning of the individual's mind or brain? *(The impairment may be a result of a condition, illness or external factors, such as alcohol or poisoning.)*

If NO, presume they have capacity; if YES, go to Stage 2

Stage 2: Is the impairment or disturbance sufficient that the individual lacks the capacity to make a specific decision?

The individual **must demonstrate all four functions** to be assessed as **having capacity:**

1. **Understand** information significant to the decision.

2. **Retain** information significant to the decision, there and then in the assessment.

3. **Weigh** up significant information and what the choices are in relation to that specific decision.

4. **Communicate** their decision to the assessor.

*The patient is usually asked to communicate the decision **back to the assessor** to show understanding.*

Determining best interests

When determining what is in the person's best interests, respect must be shown to their physical, psychological, social, ethical, spiritual and cultural being (DH, 2007).

- The person must be involved in the decision-making as much as possible.
- Establish the individual's wishes and feelings.
- Identify people who know the person.
- Avoid making the decision where possible, if the individual may regain capacity *(remember: lack of capacity may be transient and treatable, e.g. hypoxia or poisoning)*.
- Choose the least restrictive option.

Never make a decision based on a person's age, appearance, condition or behaviour/manner.

Never make a decision concerning treatment that is driven by a desire to end a person's life.

7.5 MAKING A DECISION ON BEHALF OF SOMEONE

The 'least restrictive' option

When an individual lacks the capacity to make a decision, a person may be identified to make that decision, or act on behalf of that person. Prior to identifying such a person, you must question whether there is a need to act or make the decision at all. Review whether an alternative can be found that is less restrictive on the individual's rights and freedoms; this is called the *'least restrictive option'*.

An advanced decision

An advanced decision (AD), sometimes known as a *'living will'* or an advance decision to refuse treatment (ADRT), is **legally binding** and allows a person to officially record medical treatments that the person does not want to be given in the future. They are used by individuals in case they later become incapacitated and are unable to make, or communicate, decisions. Always ensure there is proof of an AD and conditions are in place to ensure validity (see *Box 7.6*).

> ### *Box 7.6* Conditions required for an advanced decision (AD)
>
> - A person must be 18 years old or above to make an AD.
> - A person must have capacity to make the specific decision at the time the AD was made.
> - An AD can only be used if it is applicable to the actual circumstance.
>
> *Just because a 30-year-old has an AD stating that they wish to be cared for in a hospice at the end of their life, this does not necessarily mean that they wish to live in a nursing home if they were to have a sudden stroke aged 31 years.*
>
> - An AD should clearly state that the decision will still apply in life-threatening situations.
> - An AD must always be written, signed and witnessed.
>
> *If you have any doubts about the authenticity of documents, always take legal advice.*

An Advanced '*Statement*', as opposed to Advanced '*Decision*', is different as it is not legally binding; however, it can be used to guide someone who has to make a best interests decision. Statements usually detail the person's preferences, ranging from how they shave to whether they want active treatment if incapacitated in the future.

Independent mental capacity advocate

An independent mental capacity advocate (IMCA) provides representation to make a specific decision for the person who lacks capacity. The appointment of an IMCA is considered if:

- a person has no friends or relatives
- serious medical treatment is planned
- a long-term accommodation move is planned.

Lasting power of attorney

Any adult who **has mental capacity** to make the decision can grant a lasting power of attorney (LPA) to another person, or group of people, to enable them to make decisions on their behalf. Separate legal documents are usually required for different decisions. If there are disputes between appointed attorneys, or between attorneys and medical staff, the Court of

Protection will attempt to resolve disagreements. Disputes may relate to dilemmas such as whether to withdraw a particular treatment or whether or not a person is being deprived of their liberty.

If a patient does not have the capacity to make a decision, and there is no LPA with the authority to make the decision or an AD, you must check whether there is a court deputy appointed with the authority to decide. If the decision relates to serious medical treatment or a change of accommodation, then all people involved in the person's care will usually make the decision; this usually takes place in a best interests meeting. As a student or newly qualified nurse it is helpful to attend as many meetings as you can as an observer, to prepare you for future meetings.

7.6 THE IMPORTANCE OF DOCUMENTATION AND FOLLOW-UP

When a person declines care it is **essential that your documentation records your actions to promote adherence with the prescribed interventions to safeguard the person** at the time of the event and in the future. Good documentation will assure care and prevent the risk of future litigation. You must follow up with appropriate interventions and referrals in the future, which will be defined by national and local policies and procedures.

As a student or new starter, you may come across patient notes and care plans that detail conversations recorded between professionals and patients. Try to review how the narrative is recorded after a patient declines care. It is often documented verbatim in precise detail according to the facts at the time (see examples in *Boxes 6.2, 6.3* and *6.4*). The records you keep when a patient declines care should specify details according to the actual timeline at the time, and should include the following:

- Reasons for the person/significant others declining care or why you think the person is not adhering to prescribed care, if they cannot communicate this. *Do not write emotive comments of what you think are the reasons for refusal. Write facts, e.g. the patient stated he was not happy to take his medication as it makes him 'feel sick'.*

- Outcome of a mental capacity assessment for the specific decision, if indicated.

- Strategies used to overcome communication barriers and their evaluation, alternatives offered to the person and their adherence to or refusal of these options.

- Risks of non-adherence and benefits of adherence given to the person/relevant others (usually written verbatim in care plans and medical notes).

- Actions taken by staff following a patient declining or agreeing to interventions.

- Decision made by the patient/significant others, following the above interventions.

- Risk assessments completed, e.g. falls risk assessment.

- Additional use of procedural paperwork if indicated, e.g. self-discharge or DoLS forms.

- Escalation to others, according to local escalation pathway. Incident reporting may be required if adherence cannot be achieved.

- Safeguards put in place to prevent future harm to the person and/or others at risk.

- Rationale for future DoLS if indicated.

- Next of kin/relevant others informed of situation and their perspective.

- Follow-up and referrals made for future support.

REFERENCES

Department of Health (2005a) *Mental Capacity Act*. London: HMSO. Available at www.legislation.gov.uk/ukpga/2005/9 (last accessed 10 July 2018)

Department of Health (2005b) *Mental Capacity Act 2005 Deprivation of Liberty Safeguards. A guide for family, friends and unpaid carers*. London: The Stationery Office.

Department of Health (2007) *Mental Health Act 2007*. London: The Stationery Office. Available at: www.legislation.gov.uk/ukpga/2007/12/pdfs/ukpga_20070012_en.pdf (last accessed 10 July 2018)

Department of Health (2012) *Transforming Care: a national response to Winterbourne View Hospital: Department of Health Review Final Report*. London: The Stationery Office. Available at: www.gov.uk/government/uploads/system/uploads/attachment_data/file/213215/final-report.pdf (last accessed 10 July 2018)

Department of Health (2014) *Positive and Proactive Care: reducing the need for restrictive interventions*. London: Stationery Office. Available at: www.gov.uk/government/uploads/system/uploads/attachment_data/file/300293/JRA_DoH_Guidance_on_RP_web_accessible.pdf (last accessed 10 July 2018)

Northern Ireland Assembly (2016) *Mental Capacity Act (Northern Ireland) 2016*. Norwich: Stationery Office. Available at: www.legislation.gov.uk/nia/2016/18/pdfs/nia_20160018_en.pdf (last accessed 10 July 2018)

Nursing and Midwifery Council (2018) *Future Nurse: standards of proficiency for registered nurses*. Available at: www.nmc.org.uk/globalassets/sitedocuments/education-standards/future-nurse-proficiencies.pdf (accessed 19 July 2018)

Oxford English Dictionary (2018) *Oxford English Dictionary*. Oxford University Press: Oxford.

Scottish Parliament (2000) *Adults with Incapacity (Scotland) Bill*. Edinburgh: Stationery Office. Available at: www.parliament.scot/S1_Bills/Adults%20with%20Incapacity%20(Scotland)%20Bill/b5s1.pdf (last accessed 10 July 2018)

UK House of Lords (1991) *United Kingdom House of Lords Decisions: In re: F Respondent*. F v. West Berkshire Health Authority [1989] 2 AER 545 Health Authority.

WHAT TO DO NEXT

1. Discuss with your preceptor issues relating to consent, assessment of mental capacity and ethical decision-making specific to your practice area.

2. Review key national and local policies and guidelines relating to individual consent, the declining of care and advanced decisions.

3. Ask experienced colleagues what strategies they use to promote adherence and concordance and learn how to deal with the refusal of care from good role models.

4. Ask your preceptor for a copy of the local policy, protocol and clinical pathways relating to mental capacity assessments and DoLS applications.

5. Check where DoLS application forms and self-discharge forms are stored in your practice area for your future reference – often you need forms quickly and it is stressful if you have no idea.

6. Become familiar with local restraint policies and always keep up to date with national and professional standards relevant to the use of restraint in your practice area.

7. Ask your preceptor whether you need to attend specialist restraint training as part of your new role.

CHAPTER 8

UNDERSTANDING ESCALATION AND INCIDENT REPORTING

> ❝ *I learnt to take patients' obs and chart them when I was a student. If a patient's obs were too high, or low, my mentor escalated them to a doctor. I had to phone a doctor once about a patient because he was spiking a temperature, but usually mentors bleeped the doctors. They are accountable at the end of the day and now I'm qualified I'm responsible for escalation. We use NEWS and have a trigger score to tell a doctor how poorly the patient is. NEWS lets you know how often you should do your obs. You need to check the escalation pathways and tools used in your area when you start. Find out which teams to bleep too, and what numbers they're on. You might need a second opinion quickly and knowing this can save a life.* ❞

1 year post-qualified adult nurse

> ❝ *I had to write an incident form in my first month qualified. A lady with dementia was admitted with bruises over both arms. Her husband was in his 80s and they had a live-in carer. It looked like someone could have grabbed her arms but we weren't sure. The doctor told me to fill in an incident form and he took photos for her notes. He told me I couldn't presume this lady was grabbed, as I had written that she may have 'grab marks on her arms'. I needed to write just what I saw, 'bilateral bruising'. I knew if someone had bilateral bruising that cannot be accounted for, it may be a safeguarding issue. We found out later that her husband and carers were not using a hoist to transfer, as the lady hated the hoist and she was on warfarin and bruised easily. Our incident report led to managers*

educating carers and her husband about safe manual handling. It's important to escalate to a safeguarding lead to properly investigate potential issues. 〝

18 months post-qualified, community setting

Knowing how to escalate a patient's deteriorating condition, and report incidents that may cause serious harm, is an important part of a qualified nurse's role. If a deteriorating condition or untoward event is not escalated in time, to the correct person, it can impact patient outcomes or mortality rates. If you miss important observations, or signs that a patient is deteriorating, your NMC registration could be at risk. As a new starter, you need to know the details of your local escalation policy, and adhere to strict escalation pathways and standards when reporting incidents from practice. You will be expected to use your communication skills to attempt to de-escalate any challenging situations you may come across; this is sometimes termed *'conflict resolution'*.

Newly qualified nurses' concerns usually relate to three key questions: *"How do I decide if a person's situation needs to be escalated, and how do I escalate?"*, *"How do I report an incident or safeguarding issue?"* and *"How do I de-escalate a situation that is becoming difficult?"*. This chapter attempts to answer these questions, offering practical advice if you are confronted with challenging situations, or need to escalate and report incidents.

8.1 PATIENT DETERIORATION AND ESCALATION

Nurses' clinical judgement is fundamental to influencing the quality of patient care, and is based on observed and experiential data collected from patients or practice environments.

As a trained nurse you are accountable for your clinical judgements and decisions when you act, or fail to act, in practice (NMC, 2015). Clinical deterioration can happen at any stage during a patient's illness; however, patients are more susceptible after surgery and following an emergency admission or critical illness. You should continually assess and monitor patients for signs of deterioration, as part of the nursing process, and respond promptly to keep them comfortable and safe from harm (see *Section 5.2* for more on how to prioritise care).

In the past, decisions to escalate deteriorating patients relied mainly on nurses' clinical judgement. If unsure, junior nurses deferred clinical decisions to the ward sister/charge nurse or doctors. Nurse training was task-orientated; for example, I was taught to know what observations were required for specific conditions; which signs would indicate acute deterioration; how often nursing interventions should be performed; and when to escalate to medics. The development of my nursing knowledge culminated in a condition-based finals exam at the end of our course. The absence of critical appraisal and reflection within my nurse training meant I lacked the skills to question the evidence underpinning practice. We were trained '*to do*', as opposed to proactively change or influence. Ideally nurse training should aim to provide a balance between the two.

Evidence suggests that newly qualified nurses can find clinical decision-making challenging when responding to deteriorating patients (Purling and King, 2012). Nowadays, clinical guidelines, policies and standards are provided by employers to ensure staff recognise and manage acutely unwell patients according to defined escalation pathways. Clinical escalation in your local area should reflect current NICE guidelines, relating to assessing and managing acute illness in adults (NICE, 2007); common mental health problems and pathways to care (NICE, 2011); fever in children under the age of five (NICE, 2017); and bronchiolitis in children (NICE, 2015a).

The need to recognise acutely ill and deteriorating patients

The creation of prescriptive escalation standards and early warning systems (EWS) arose from reports of adverse events across the NHS. A need was identified to improve patient safety and clinical outcomes which, in turn, would decrease the potential for future litigation. National evidence identified that deterioration of patients in acute hospital settings occasionally went undetected and harmful clinical events were attributed to errors in clinical judgement. In 2005, The National Patient Safety Agency (NPSA) examined 576 hospital deaths over one year and found that 11% were due to deterioration '*not being recognised*' or '*acted upon*' (NPSA, 2007). It was estimated that approximately 23 000 hospital deaths per year in the UK due to cardiac arrest could have been avoided with better observations and escalation processes. Poorer patient outcomes and higher mortality rates were linked to vital physiological observations not being recorded often enough or not being recognised as abnormal (Hillman *et al.*, 2001; NPSA, 2007; National Confidential Enquiry into Patient Outcome and Death, 2005; Smith *et al.*, 2006).

Patient deterioration may not be detected because it has **not been recognised,** due to inadequate observation or clinical assessment. This may happen because of:

- staff lacking adequate knowledge as to how often to perform observations/clinical assessments
- staff not recognising the parameters for normal/abnormal patient observations
- patient giving inaccurate information to staff
- patient being nursed in a side room, or behind curtains, leading to signs being missed
- staff lacking experience in managing acutely ill patients
- staff unable to correctly set alarm parameters on monitoring equipment
- out-of-date monitoring equipment, e.g. blood glucose reading inaccurately
- care plans out of date or incorrect nursing interventions
- prescribed medical care incorrect or mistakenly interpreted, e.g. poor handwriting
- inadequate nursing handover of observations required
- workload and patient dependencies too high and staff unable to perform observations on time
- nurse unable to manage time/feeling overwhelmed by work allocated
- incompetent and/or lazy staff.

Deterioration of patients may alternatively not be detected because it has **not been acted on,** due to poor communication and escalation. This may happen because of:

- staff lacking knowledge of local escalation policies, procedures and standards
- inadequate/incorrect use of early warning systems
- unclear verbal escalation by staff
- poor communication/relations between nursing and medical teams, leading to absence of response following escalation.

How to recognise and respond to acute illness

It is evident that early recognition, timely escalation and a competent clinical response will determine the clinical outcomes of individuals with acute illness. To promote prompt recognition of deterioration and responsive treatment for acutely ill adults in hospital, NICE has issued key guidelines and evidence-based recommendations (NICE, 2007); these are summarised in *Table 8.1*).

Table 8.1: Summary of recommendations for acutely ill adults in hospital (NICE, 2007)

Key area	Evidence-based recommendations
Observations	Observations recorded at time of admission or initial assessment
	Minimum physiological observations recorded include: heart rate; respiratory rate; blood pressure; level of consciousness, oxygen saturation and temperature
	Observations monitored at least every 12 hours, unless a decision made at a senior level to increase/decrease frequency
	In specific circumstances, additional monitoring considered, e.g. hourly urine output or pain assessment
Written plan	A written monitoring plan specifying which observations recorded and how often; plans take account of patients' diagnosis, comorbidities and agreed treatments
Identify deterioration/risk of deterioration	Track and trigger systems monitor all adult patients in acute settings, such as multiple-parameter or aggregate weighted scoring systems, to allow a graded response
	Frequency of monitoring increased if abnormal physiology detected
Trained staff to act upon observations	Observations recorded and acted upon by staff trained to undertake them and understand their relevance
	Staff caring for patients in acute hospital settings competent in monitoring, measurement, interpretation and prompt response
	Education and training provided to ensure staff can demonstrate competence
Transfer of patients	Decision to transfer patients from wards to critical care, and vice versa, involves consultants from both areas
	Transfer from critical care areas to the general ward avoided between 22.00 and 07.00 if possible
	Critical care and ward teams take shared responsibility for the care of the patient being transferred, to ensure continuity and structured handover of care

National Early Warning Score (NEWS)

The use of early warning scores (EWS), to help detect a patient's deterioration and advise prompt medical escalation, was first recommended by the Department of Health in their publication *Comprehensive Critical Care: a review of adult critical care services* (DH, 2000). The National Early Warning Score (NEWS) was initially developed in 2012 by the Royal College of Physicians to improve the detection of, and response to clinical deterioration in adult patients in UK acute hospital settings (RCP, 2012).

The original NEWS tool was updated in 2017 to NEWS2, incorporating the needs of patients with sepsis and renewing physiological parameters (RCP, 2017). NICE (2007) recommends the use of physiological *'track and trigger'* systems to monitor all adult patients in acute hospital settings. NHS Improvement is requesting 100% use of NEWS2 in acute and ambulance settings by March 2019.

A range of EWS have been modified to meet the needs of specific patient types:

Paediatric Early Warning Score (PEWS) (Monaghan, 2005)

- Its goal is to improve early recognition and management of seriously ill/deteriorating children less than 16 years old.
- Children have different normal ranges for observations than adults.

Modified Early Obstetric Warning Score (MEOWS) (Lewis, 2007)

- Its goal is to improve early recognition/management of seriously ill/deteriorating women receiving care from maternity services.
- MEOWS covers physiological parameters/changes required for pregnant women.

Modified Early Warning Score (MEWS) (Subbe *et al.*, 2001; NCEPOD, 2005)

- Its goal is to improve early recognition of seriously ill/deteriorating people in various clinical situations, such as adult patients attending specialist areas, day surgery units and outpatients.
- There is evidence of use in mental health and learning disability settings.

National Early Warning Score (NEWS2) (RCP, 2017)

- Its goal is to improve early recognition of seriously ill/deteriorating adults in acute and ambulance settings.
- NEWS incorporates the needs of patients with sepsis.

How does 'track and trigger' work?

Early warning scores (EWS) are used as part of a track and trigger system to alert staff to clinically deteriorating adults or children. EWS are used to quickly establish a level of illness for a patient, i.e. how poorly, or at risk of deterioration the person is. The track and trigger system combines a patient's observation chart with an early warning scoring system, to record a total EWS. The total track and trigger score, or EWS, will indicate whether a patient is stable and at low risk of deterioration, indicated by a low score; or very poorly with a high risk of deterioration, indicated by a triggering high score.

The EWS system relies on the nurse performing intermittent physiological observations and assessments that are scored to track a patient's condition. Predetermined normal/abnormal parameters are related to each observation; for example, normal blood pressure will score 0 and hypertension may score 3. Each individual score is added up on a track and trigger chart and a total EWS awarded.

The NEWS2 for adults combines scores from six physiological parameters. There is one additional weighted score for supplemental oxygen. NEWS2 scores relating to normal/abnormal physiological observations are presented in *Table 8.2*, according to current NEWS2 (RCP, 2017) guidance.

How should you respond to your total early warning score?

It is important to remember that you must view the person as a whole and not just a set of signs and symptoms when using any EWS. Clinical deterioration can be identified through changes to several observations or a great change to one clinical observation/assessment. An urgent escalation may be prompted, even if the person's physiological observations are not triggering a response, e.g. when a patient is expressing suicidal thoughts; is in severe pain; has reduced urine output or is unable to swallow and presenting with dehydration.

The response to EWS is guided by your local policy and escalation standards/pathways that should be informed by NICE guidelines (NICE, 2007). You must identify and review local escalation procedures and tools used when you start in a new practice setting. Throughout your career, you need to adhere to future changes, as escalation pathways are regularly updated according to the latest evidence base. Senior nurses should observe you completing track and trigger charts to ensure you are competent and they can advise as needed.

Table 8.2: National Early Warning Score 2 (NEWS2) for adult observations (RCP, 2017)

NEWS2 observations	Parameters	Track and trigger score
Respiratory rate (respirations per minute)	≥25	3
	21–24	2
	12–20	0
	9–11	1
	≤8	3
Oxygen saturation **Note:** target ranges are different if hypercapnic or respiratory failure	≥96%	0
	94–95%	1
	92–93%	2
	≤91%	3
Systolic blood pressure (mmHg)	≥220	3
	111–219	0
	101–110	1
	91–100	2
	51–90	3
	≤50	3
Pulse rate (beats per minute)	≥131	3
	111–130	2
	91–110	1
	51–90	0
	41–50	1
	31–40	3
	≤30	3
Level of consciousness / new confusion (AVPU / GCS (Glasgow Coma Scale))	Alert	0
	Confusion	3
	Voice	3
	Pain	3
	Unresponsive	3
Temperature	≥39.1°C	2
	38.1–39°C	1
	36.1–38°C	0
	35.1–36°C	3
	≤35°C	3

NOTE: *Example physiological parameters shown reflect RCP (2017) guidance; however, parameters can differ according to your speciality. The highlighted scores are optimal.*

What is an escalation pathway?

An escalation pathway will be activated when a maximum threshold, or trigger level, for the total EWS is reached. Each trigger level on a pathway will prescribe:

- how often clinical monitoring / observations should be performed
- the minimum time frame for medical review
- the qualification of the person undertaking the review.

The RCP (2017) recommends three NEWS2 trigger levels for a clinical alert, defined as low, medium or high. Defined trigger levels are detailed within local escalation pathways, standards or procedures. Current RCP (2017) guidelines suggest the following for adults in acute care settings:

- **LOW NEWS2** total score (0):
  - continue routine monitoring
  - frequency of monitoring – **minimum 12-hourly**
- **LOW NEWS2** total score (1–4):
  - assessment by a competent registered nurse: RN decides whether to increase frequency and/or escalate further
  - frequency of monitoring – **minimum 4–6-hourly**
- **MEDIUM URGENT RESPONSE NEWS2** total score (5–6, or a score of 3 in one parameter):
  - RN to immediately inform medical team and prompt urgent review by a clinician competent to assess acute illness, usually a ward-based doctor or senior specialist nurse, provide clinical care in an environment with monitoring facilities
  - frequency of monitoring – **minimum 1-hourly**
- **HIGH EMERGENCY RESPONSE NEWS2** total scores (≥7):
  - RN to inform medical team immediately, at least at specialist registrar level – emergency assessment by team with critical care competencies includes practitioner with advanced airway management skills; transfer care to a level 2/3 clinical care facility, e.g. high dependency unit or ICU
  - frequency of monitoring – **continuous monitoring of vital signs.**

As well as numeric triggers, EWS charts are colour-coded as red, amber and green / blue to provide visual prompts for abnormal clinical parameters.

RCP (2017) NEWS2 colour codes advising the monitoring of adults within acute care settings are presented as follows:

- ≥7 total NEWS2 = **RED**: continuous monitoring of vital signs
- 5–7 total NEWS2 = **AMBER**: increase frequency to a minimum of 1-hourly
- 1–4 total NEWS2 = **GREEN**: minimum 4–6-hourly
- 0 = **BLUE**: 6–12-hourly

Do I need training to use EWS systems?

You must be trained, and assessed as competent, before using any EWS systems employed in a practice area (NICE, 2007; RCP, 2017). Many practice areas provide local training for new starter nurses, such as competency skills-based training or 'recognising acutely ill and deteriorating patients' (RAID) courses. Ask your line manager or preceptor the following questions:

- **What EWS system and escalation pathways/standards are used in this area?**
- **What training/escalation competencies do you expect me to achieve?**
- **What are time frames for achievement?**
- **What courses are available for me to book?**
- **Who will assess my competence to use EWS?**

If you have limited experience working in acute care settings, or you are working in specialist care, you may require additional training; for example, to perform a GCS assessment or use equipment, such as monitors. Experienced nurses will advise on the training required to demonstrate competent use of assessments and equipment.

Communication aids to cascade information

When escalating an EWS trigger score, you must cascade information to the relevant professional. Many NHS trusts expect staff to use standardised communication models to promote clear communications and assurance that the information cascaded is correct. Popular handover tools use simple mnemonics to aid communication, such as **SBAR** (Pope *et al.*,

2008) or **RSVP** (Featherstone *et al.*, 2008), presented in *Tables 8.3* and *8.4*, respectively. Always check whether a specific model is being used in practice and ensure you are trained to competently complete the forms and verbally cascade information. Remember that mnemonic handover aids provide an important record of cascaded data that is kept in patients' notes.

Table 8.3: Example SBAR communication aid (Pope et al., 2008)

Mnemonic	Example prompts	Extracts of example text
SITUATION	Your name, role and title State the problem (time when started) and what is happening now	"Staff Nurse X on Y ward. Rang Dr W Senior Registrar. Mr Z had sudden severe abdominal pain since 8am that has not improved over last 10 minutes. Mr Z states he cannot bear the pain any more and has been screaming in pain."
BACKGROUND	Clear / concise relevant past medical history Reason for admission	"Mr Z is a 20-year-old male, admitted for a routine outpatient appointment. He was sat in our outpatients when he bent up double and suddenly called out in pain. No relevant medical history apart from tingling in foot. He was waiting in outpatients to see neurologist."
ASSESSMENT	Observations / clinical assessment ABCDE assessment Track and trigger score	"Vital signs carried at [date / time] by the nurse: BP 130/90; P 90, oxygen saturations 98% , etc; Track &Trigger score X; Mr Z has no problems breathing and is fully orientated. Mr Z has no rashes but complains of extreme lower abdominal pain. He stated that he has never experienced pain like this before."
RECOMMENDATIONS	Request recommendation from doctor Plan for review by doctor	"Dr W requested that Mr Z is immediately placed on bed in outpatients and nurse must stay with patient until he arrives. Dr W will review Mr Z immediately. In the meantime nurses to conduct 15 minutes observations, continuous monitoring and ECG."

Table 8.4: Example RSVP communication aid (Featherstone et al., 2008)

Mnemonic	Example prompts
REASON	Caller's name / role
	Location: ward X
	Patient's name, DOB
	Location of patient
	Check name of person you are speaking to and their role
STORY	Background information and what is happening
	Past medical history and reason for admission
	DNR status / other information
VITAL SIGNS	Vital signs
	Prescribed oxygen therapy
	Urine output, fluid balance, changes to bowel output, excessive sweating
	Pain assessment score
	Track and trigger score
PLAN	What you have done so far and plan to do
	Support requested and action
	What you think is required from person

8.2 INCIDENT REPORTING

The majority of nurses have to report untoward incidents during their career and these will require the recording of events on a clinical incident form. Examples of potential situations that may be escalated and recorded are presented in *Box 8.1*.

When dealing with a reportable incident, your initial priorities should be as follows:

1. **Safety:** avoid putting yourself or others at risk when dealing with incidents. Ensure patients/staff/others are safe at all times; for example, take items out of a confused person's reach to prevent them injuring themselves or others.

2. **Escalation:** escalate to senior nurses or doctors (as per escalation pathway) and request support from appropriate teams who can advise on additional strategies.

Box 8.1 Potential situations escalated and recorded on an incident form

- Patient and staff injuries, e.g. slips, trips and falls; newly acquired pressure ulcers, and needlestick injuries.

- Care issue that compromises patient / staff safety, e.g. safeguarding issues or lack of resources.

- Errors, e.g. medication administration errors, including medications being missed and patient non-adherence.

- Untoward events, e.g. a confused patient who cannot be found.

- System / procedure failure, e.g. patient's discharge cancelled due to lack of adequate support.

- Equipment failures, e.g. IV insulin being administered too quickly.

- Aggressive behaviour by patients / others (includes verbal aggression).

- Problems with working environment, e.g. heating broken down.

- Human error, e.g. air cylinder brought to a cardiac arrest instead of oxygen.

- Complaints made by patients, significant others, and other health care professionals.

3. **Reporting and recording:** report and record events on a clinical incident form along with actions taken at the time. Actions and interventions relating to a patient care incident must be recorded in care plan and medical notes too.

Following escalation and the recording of an incident, data from the report will be investigated and analysed by your line manager / employer to plan for improvements within the service. The follow-up investigation may involve you writing more detailed statements about what happened at the time. You should always **take legal advice** from your union representatives if your performance is being formally investigated as part of an incident report (see *Chapter 9* for further details).

Professional duty of candour

It is important that your employer has an open incident reporting structure, to tackle inadequate systems and prevent future incidents. Always seek support from experienced nurses and your line manager if you have made an error or are worried about reporting an incident. Employers should be sympathetic to human error and encourage a climate of learning from mistakes, as opposed to promoting a blame culture that deters staff from reporting incidents.

The NMC and GMC (2015) advocate openness and honesty when things go wrong, as health care professionals have a professional duty of candour. These person-centred recommendations promote positive open communication and help to de-escalate a challenging nurse–patient encounter or prevent a future complaint (see the recommendations in *Box 8.2*).

Box 8.2 Professional duty of candour recommendations for health care professional (adapted from NMC and GMC, 2015)

- Be open and honest with patients when something goes wrong or has potential to cause harm.
- Be open and honest with employers / regulators, raising concerns where appropriate, and participate in reviews / investigations when requested.
- Support and encourage colleagues to be open and honest – do not stop someone from raising concerns.
- Tell the patient, or patient's family / carer when something goes wrong.
- Apologise to the patient, or patient's family / carer, when something goes wrong
- Offer appropriate solution or support / advice to make it right, if feasible for you to do so.
- Explain to the patient, or patient's family / carer, the short- and long-term effects of what has happened.

Failure to report

Failure to report an untoward incident is unacceptable and indicates *'cultural safety failings'* in an organisation, such as those reported following the Mid Staffordshire NHS Foundation Trust Public Inquiry (Francis, 2013). If you fail to escalate, report and deal with an incident appropriately (for example, when a vulnerable patient falls out of bed) and the person later comes to serious harm or dies, you may be called to court as part of a coroner's inquest. A lack of appropriate escalation and actions following a clinical incident or error may be deemed serious professional misconduct, according to the NMC *Code* (NMC, 2015).

Improving quality

Health care employers must demonstrate how their organisation intends to improve safety and quality, and reduce the risk of harm. Your line manager/employer is responsible for continually reviewing all clinical incidents that occur within their service. They must analyse information from incidents and follow up investigations and interpret data to guide their safety improvement plans.

Always seize opportunities to attend quality assurance, clinical governance or clinical incident review meetings, to increase your understanding of local quality improvement processes.

A few key terms you may come across in practice linked to quality improvement within the NHS are explained in *Table 8.5*.

National quality standards/measurements

The Care Quality Commission (CQC) has a responsibility to assess the performance of health care organisations to ensure they meet the standards required, according to key performance indicators (KPIs; see *Box 8.3* for example KPIs). NHS performance is also evaluated against population screening standards, such as breast screening and foetal anomaly screening.

Table 8.5: Key terms linked to quality improvement

Key term	Simple explanation
Clinical governance	Umbrella term: includes systems that maintain high standards, improve quality care or promote clinical excellence
	All elements within *Chapter 8* are part of *'clinical governance'* such as: escalation pathways; incident reporting; learning from mistakes; clinical audits; promoting evidence-based standards; and devising action plans following analysis of incidents/complaints
Risk management	Involves predicting and evaluating clinical risks, e.g. analysing data from clinical incidents and complaints, along with identifying strategies to avoid/minimise future risk
Quality assurance	Process of checking that defined health care standards are met
	Includes a variety of strategies, e.g. clinical audits, patient satisfaction and staff feedback surveys
Clinical audit	An evaluation of clinical service using a defined standard, e.g. a documentation audit to evaluate whether nurses adhere to record-keeping standards from the NMC (NMC, 2015)

Box 8.3 Some example key performance indicators (KPIs) (NHS England, 2016)

- Number of emergency calls abandoned after at least 30 seconds and average time to answer.
- Average time to complete urgent clinical assessments.
- Rate of compliance with medical advice.
- Number of serious incidents.
- Average time to definitive clinical encounter.
- High rates of patient satisfaction.

Never Events

'*Never Events*' are a category of incidents that are very serious and mainly preventable, and which must be publicly reported to prevent re-occurrence (NHS England, 2015; see *Box 8.4*).

Box 8.4 The Never Events list 2015/16 (NHS England, 2015)

- Wrong site surgery
- Wrong implant / prosthesis
- Retained foreign object post-procedure
- Mis-selection of strong potassium-containing solution
- Wrong route administration of medication
- Overdose of insulin due to abbreviations or incorrect device
- Overdose of methotrexate for non-cancer treatment
- Mis-selection of high strength midazolam during conscious sedation
- Failure to install functional collapsible shower or curtain rails
- Falls from poorly restricted windows
- Chest or neck entrapment in bedrails
- Transfusion or transplantation of ABO-incompatible blood components or organs
- Misplaced nasogastric or oro-gastric tubes
- Scalding of patients

After a Never Event, a formal process should be adhered to by medical/nursing leads, guided by NHS England (2015); see *Box 8.5*.

Box 8.5 After a Never Event

- Inform lead in the organisation that a Never Event has happened, according to local policy.

- Inform patient/significant other as soon as possible, following principles of *'duty of candour'*.

- Response to a Never Event coordinated by a nursing or medical director, as soon as identified.

- Lead discusses and agrees Never Event; then reports on Strategic Executive Information System. Incident reported on local risk management system within two working days of identification.

- Systematic investigation to be completed and future implementation plan to be reported.

- Report implications of Never Event at public board meeting and share learning on Strategic Executive Information System (types and numbers are written in local/national annual reports).

Monitoring performance

Performance data from NHS providers is available through national IT systems which monitor trends monthly, quarterly and annually. The public can access key performance data online for any NHS hospital. Trust board and commissioning groups also provide information relating to local provision that is readily available to employees on local intranet sites.

It is useful to review documents linked to the performance of your service, to increase your knowledge of standard setting and the future goals or initiatives planned. As a third year student, performance data may assist your decision when choosing your first job. For example, are there plans to close a department or move services elsewhere, or have they been rated as 'inadequate' during a recent CQC visit with numerous reports of Never Events?

How to record a clinical incident

Once an incident has been reported, it must be recorded, adhering to professional record-keeping standards (see *Chapter 6*). Additional pointers are presented below:

- Find out where clinical incident forms are stored and how they are completed. When completing this form for the first time, ask an experienced nurse to check your narrative.

- Language used on forms should be objective and you must only write what was witnessed at the time. Do not use an emotive style that attempts to apportion blame. Write factual accounts and direct quotes only.

- Document important details as soon after an incident as possible to recall facts, such as: times; order of events; who said what; the actions of staff at the time and after; and who witnessed the events.

- If a member of staff witnessed the incident they should be the person completing the incident form.

- If a number of witnesses were involved, then one person should take the lead to ensure someone follows through to complete the form.

- If a nurse on the prior shift witnesses an incident, they should not pass the job of completing the incident form to the next shift.

A summary of key data required on a clinical incident form is presented in *Box 8.6*.

Box 8.6 Key data required on a clinical incident form

- Patient details: full name, date of birth and hospital number
- Date, time and location of incident
- Details of the person reporting the incident: name, role and contact details
- Factual, chronological description of incident
- Details of all witnesses: full name, roles (e.g. staff, patients, relatives) and contact details
- Factual details of harm caused, if any
- Actions taken at the time, and by whom (full name and role).

Overall risk rating

Clinical incident forms use risk matrices to calculate an overall risk rating, as follows:

Consequence rating × Likelihood rating = Overall risk rating

The overall risk rating is graded to provide an impression of whether there is a *'low'* to *'extreme'* risk of re-occurrence of harm (see *Table 8.6*). Examples of risk matrices linked to *'consequences'* and *'likelihood of occurrence'* that the risk will happen again, are presented in *Tables 8.7* and *8.8*, respectively.

Table 8.6: Graded risk scores for incidents

Graded risk	Score
LOW risk	1–3
MODERATE risk	4–6
HIGH risk	8–12
EXTREME risk	15–25

Table 8.7: Consequence rating scores

Score	Type of consequence / injury
1	**Insignificant**; minimum injury; no intervention / treatment prescribed
2	**Minor** injury; minor intervention
3	**Moderate** injury requiring intervention from a professional; RIDDOR reportable
4	**Major** injury; leading to long-term incapacity; disability
5	**Catastrophic** incident leading to death

Table 8.8: Likelihood rating scores

Score	Type of consequence / injury
1	**Rare** – probably will never happen again; or not expected to occur for years
2	**Unlikely** – not expected to recur, but may be possible; expected to occur at least annually
3	**Possible** – might recur occasionally, expected to occur at least monthly
4	**Likely** – probably will recur but not continuing issue that is expected
5	**Almost certain** – will undoubtedly recur, probably frequently, expected to occur at least daily

8.3 DE-ESCALATING CHALLENGING SITUATIONS

Working in challenging health care environments means that preventing, and dealing with, interpersonal conflict is an inevitable part of your role. Conflicts do not just occur between patients / relatives and staff; conflict may need resolving between members of your team (see *Chapter 9* for further support if an issue has arisen between you and a member of staff).

Many employers offer training programmes to increase staff knowledge to defuse potential situations; this is often called conflict resolution or de-escalation training. Discuss with your preceptor potential challenging situations that may arise within your practice setting.

A person may be angry or upset, indicating that a situation may escalate, if they:

- appear agitated, raise their voice, swear or directly threaten someone
- invade another individual's personal space, or stand over someone who is sitting down
- point their fingers or increase gesticulations

- start to pace up and down, clench their fists or stiffen their body
- appear frightened, confused or disorientated
- smell of alcohol or show signs of drug use, e.g. pinpoint pupils/slurred speech
- are violent, throw objects or attempt to push/punch people or throw things.

When you start in post, be proactive and ready to deal with challenging situations before they arise (see key pointers in *Box 8.7*).

Box 8.7 Key pointers to be proactive

- Never put yourself or others at risk. Always ask for help from colleagues, senior staff and/or medics when dealing with unpredictable situations.

- Whenever there are signs that a person or situation has the potential to escalate, you should call for help **earlier rather than later.**

- Establish what security is available to you and the correct numbers to contact. In any hospital/institution environment there should be on-call security and a bleep system for emergencies. Many reception areas have security numbers near to phones and/or placed on back of staff ID cards.

- In a community setting adhere to lone working policies and individual emergency call systems if doing home visits.

- In any working environment, the police can be called if situations become dangerous/out of control.

How to deal with complaints

The majority of complaints in practice can be dealt with using good listening skills and open communication. Usually complaints start off as a simple question or problem, but can quickly escalate if they are not handled empathetically and professionally at the time. Pointers that may help you deal with complaints, and de-escalate potential situations, are presented in *Table 8.9*.

Table 8.9: Strategies to deal with complaints

Key area	Pointers
Establish the issue	Give the person your name and role, and state you are there to help them (see the #hellomynameis campaign online).
	Establish why the person is complaining and try to put yourself in their shoes, e.g. are they grieving or have they had an operation cancelled more than once?
	Talk to the person complaining in a quiet place with seating and not at a busy desk with lots of commotion.
Listen and acknowledge the complaint	Genuinely listen to what the person is saying, acknowledge their complaint and try to put it right, with realistic timelines for goals.
	Do not offer to sort problems out if you have no means to do so. Often complaints escalate when the person feels let down. Do not say that you will inform the doctor and then not do this, or that you will be back in 5 minutes and not return.
	Apologise, if the person has a valid complaint, e.g. *"I am very sorry you feel that the care has been poor – shall we discuss your concerns in the quiet room to plan how we can improve the situation?"*
	A written apology from the service manager should be given if it is recognised that something has gone wrong. Usually the patient and their family / significant others will have a chance to discuss their complaint with the key service lead.
Use an open, honest and sympathetic approach	Use clear language and avoid medical jargon.
	Use open language and posture that suggests an honest and sympathetic approach, which is more likely to result in a positive experience for all.
	Give the person your undivided attention and never be confrontational, e.g. do not answer back in annoyance and raise your voice.
Escalate to others	If you cannot resolve a problem or complaint quickly, escalate to your seniors.
	Ensure you adhere to local complaints policy.
	Focus on problem-solving and avoid passing the buck or blaming others.
Help the person if they wish to formally complain	Advise a patient / family to complain formally through the Patient Advice and Liaison Service (PALS) or give them the name / contact details of lead manager / head of service. Information should come from one lead to prevent conflicting information.
	The local policy for managing complaints should be adhered to and the complainant should also have a copy.
Document and record	Make a record of what happened, what you said and any actions taken, using the clinical incident reporting system.
	If indicated, record in patient and/or medical notes.

Table 8.9: (Continued)

Key area	Pointers
If person is aggressive, escalate and ask for support	Do not take the complaint personally, as whoever is dealing with this person will receive the same treatment as you.
	If the person uses a threatening manner, inform them that you cannot talk to them while they are shouting at you and disengage from the conversation.
	Remain calm and keep stating that you will come back to talk to them when they have calmed down or they can visit PALS.
	Never go into a quiet room on your own with a person who is showing signs of aggression, even if they have calmed down and you feel safe. Ask another member of staff to be present with you and leave the door open, or talk to them in a public space.
	If you find yourself in a room with the person, position yourself / staff near to the door to prevent anyone barricading you in.
	If the person does not calm down after using suggested strategies, call security and escalate to senior (see *Box 8.7*).
	Adhere to HR policies and guidelines to support any bullying and harassment and zero tolerance for aggression towards staff.

8.4 HOW TO DEAL WITH A PATIENT'S DEATH AND A DECEASED BODY

Wherever you work, you may have to deal with a patient's death at some point during your career; such a death may be sudden or unexpected. Caring for a person who is near to death, or has died, is a privilege and requires key communication skills, compassion and empathy. Dealing with a patient death for the first time can feel daunting and a team approach should always be used to ensure the person caring for a patient's deceased body and their next of kin feel supported. Patient allocation and caseloads should be reconfigured to allow staff time to care for the patient's body respectfully and calmly. Often colleagues will offer to stay on after shifts to support you and help prepare the body, prior to removal to a mortuary or home.

Care of the dying and end of life care is a whole specialist area in itself and there are numerous national educational programmes and books you can read to increase your knowledge. It is helpful to review related NICE clinical guidelines, such as *NG31: Care of Dying Adults in the Last Days of Life* (NICE, 2015b) and *NG61: End of Life Care for Infants, Children and Young People with Life-limiting Conditions: planning and management* (NICE, 2016). When you qualify, look out for *'end of life'* study days and *'care of the dying'* short courses delivered by local hospices and oncology units that are often free to nursing staff.

Numerous students find that they have never experienced a death by the time they qualify and worry about how they will cope when they have to deal with the death of one of their patients in the future. Even if you have experienced a patient death during your training, you may need to revisit key standards and policies when you qualify, relating to administrative responsibilities, how to care for the body after death and supporting relatives of the deceased. A few of the common questions nurses ask are shown below, along with pointers to guide you.

What should happen when a patient's death is imminent?

- Identify the patient's wishes and aim to meet their individual needs and requests, e.g. if they wish to die at home.

- Maintain a calm, quiet and professional atmosphere around the patient.

- When death is imminent, re-allocate caseloads and patient allocations to allow the named nurse to provide 1:1 patient care and/or offer them additional nursing assistant support.

- Aim for continuity of staff on rotas to ensure the same team of nurses care for the patient and next of kin, where possible.

- When a patient is near to death, care for them in a comfortable quiet hospital/hospice side room or a room of their choosing at home. Make appropriate provision for relatives to stay near to the patient if requested, e.g. provide a reclining chair/camp bed in a side room or near site accommodation.

- Identify any religious requests/requirements, as you may need to contact local faith representatives.

- Next of kin should be kept informed about deterioration in the patient's condition, in line with patient's wishes.

- Offer meetings between clinicians and next of kin to answer questions.

- Establish if next of kin wish to be called in the middle of the night or not. Some may wish to sit with the patient if death is imminent and may become very distressed if not present during death. Others will be unhappy if called during unsocial hours.

- Always ensure you have the **correct next of kin contact phone numbers** and establish who should be called first if the patient's condition deteriorates. It can cause a great deal of stress if you do not have the correct telephone numbers or you phone an ex-spouse by accident.

- Look after the next of kin just as much as the patient, as they may be very stressed about the situation. Offer regular tea and coffee and support them by offering breaks, e.g. sitting with the patient.

- If next of kin cannot be present, you must communicate clearly according to the patient's wishes and offer phone discussions with the medical team.

How is a person's death confirmed?

- A death must always be formally assessed, confirmed and recorded in the patient's notes by a registered medical practitioner. Nursing staff should inform the doctor and request that death is confirmed and certified.

- **A medical certificate of cause of death book must be completed by the registered medic.** When you start in practice, find out where this book and death certificates are kept.

- If a district nurse or an out-of-hours doctor verifies a death in the community overnight, you will need to obtain a medical certificate of cause of death from the GP the next day.

- Following a patient's death, always adhere to local employer *'death and dying'* policies and procedures.

- When certifying a death in hospital, medics must identify the patient using their wrist band. In the community, next of kin must provide formal ID if the GP does not know the patient. Date, time of death and deceased state of a person must be recorded.

- It is normal for a patient's breathing to gradually decrease to a few breaths per minute when death is near, which leads to apnoea (called Cheyne–Stokes breathing). It is not unheard of for patients to be breathing when a medic arrives to confirm death, as the nurse did not observe apnoea long enough. Clinicians should listen for a lack of heart and breathing sounds for five minutes to establish cardiorespiratory arrest has occurred (timings may vary between employers and local policies).

- Ideally next of kin are present during death. If not, the nurse must inform next of kin of the death and provide them with adequate support and clear information, e.g. where to collect property, where the deceased patient will be placed and who to contact if they wish to view the body.

What happens after death?

- Last offices are carried out according to your employer procedures (see local procedures/policy).

- In hospitals/institutions, always store and record patient property in line with employer policies, e.g. two staff check property items into a property book. Ask an experienced nurse to observe you completing the property book when it is your first time.

- If death occurs in hospital, patient notes will be retained along with notification forms for the bereavement officer to collect.

- Next of kin will obtain the patient's death certificate from the bereavement office.

- Similarly, in the community case notes are retained and death must be formally recorded. The next of kin will need to obtain the medical certificate from the GP to register the death and arrange the funeral.

- Nurses are responsible for completing a bereavement service notification form and leaving messages with the bereavement office.

- Nurses contact porters to move a deceased body to a mortuary. The body will usually be kept in the hospital mortuary until the funeral directors or next of kin arrange otherwise, e.g. the body to be taken home or to a chapel of rest.

- In the community the next of kin arrange to transport the deceased body, e.g. to a funeral parlour.

- A person's death must be registered within 5 days in England, Wales or Northern Ireland and within 8 days in Scotland. Appropriate ID must be shown to register a death.

- A death is registered in the following offices:
  - England and Wales: the register office
  - Northern Ireland: the district registration office
  - Scotland: the registrar of births, deaths and marriages.

- A coroner's inquest is a legal inquiry into a death when the cause is unknown, violent or 'unnatural'. Coroner's inquests are held in public and the cause of death is determined by a coroner.
- If there is a coroner's inquest registration is delayed until the inquest is completed.

What happens during last offices (care after death)?

- Laying out a person following their death during last offices (care after death) should always be carried out with respect and professionalism.
- Always check that the patient's ID band on their wrist is legible and place another wrist band around one ankle. **The patient should always have two matching ID bands on their person.**
- You must always aim to adhere to religious/cultural rites following a person's death. It is helpful to review how different religions care for their deceased during your orientation so you are well prepared.
- Dentures should be left in place, along with a wedding ring that should be taped.
- If a wedding ring is left on the person it must be recorded in a property book in case it is reported missing later. Other jewellery is usually removed and recorded in the patient property book.
- Next of kin may later decide to remove a wedding ring; however, they must formally request this through the bereavement/property office and bring ID before they receive any patient's property.
- Usually a deceased body is washed and dentures should be replaced if they were not *in situ* at the time of death. The person should be shaved, if usual for them, and their hair brushed. Two staff members should be present during washing and last offices, to treat the body with dignity.
- There is no need to pack orifices unless there is excessive body fluid leaking out. If packs are required, orifices should be packed with gauze only.
- Soiled dressings should be redressed.
- ET tubes should be left in place if the cause of death is uncertain and referred to a coroner.
- IV lines and drains/catheters should be left *in situ* but clamped to reduce leakage.

- The patient's body is usually placed in a disposable shroud in hospital unless next of kin have requested that clothes be worn. The patient's arms are usually placed at the sides of the body within the shroud/body bag.

- The patient is usually wrapped in a clean sheet – use two sheets if the person is very large or tall.

- A Deceased Patient ID card is usually placed in a pocket on the body bag or taped to a sheet over the chest area.

- Standard infection control precautions need to be observed for all patients and appropriate personal protective equipment used, if indicated.

REFERENCES

Department of Health (2000) *Comprehensive Critical Care. A review of adult critical care services.* London: DH.

Featherstone, P., Chalmers, T. and Smith, G.B. (2008) RSVP: a system for communication of deterioration in hospital patients. *British Journal of Nursing,* **17**(13): 860–864.

Francis, R. (2013) *Report of the Mid Staffordshire NHS Foundation Trust Public Inquiry: executive summary.* London: the Stationery Office.

#hellomynameis online campaign: https://hellomynameis.org.uk/

Hillman, K.M., Bristow, P.J., Chey, T. *et al.* (2001) Antecedents to hospital deaths. *Internal Medicine Journal,* **31**(6): 343–348.

Lewis, G. (ed.) (2007) *Saving Mothers' Lives: reviewing maternal deaths to make motherhood safer 2003–2005. The seventh confidential enquiry into maternal deaths in the United Kingdom.* London: CEMACH.

Monaghan, A. (2005) Detecting and managing deterioration in children. *Paediatric Nursing,* **17**(1): 32–35.

National Confidential Enquiry into Patient Outcome and Death (2005) *An Acute Problem? A report of the National Confidential Enquiry into Patient Outcome and Death.* London: NCEPOD.

National Patient Safety Agency (2007) *Safer Care for the Acutely Ill Patient: learning from serious incidents.* London: NPSA.

NHS England (2015) *Revised Never Events Policy and Framework.* London: NHS England. Available at: www.england.nhs.uk/wp-content/uploads/2015/03/never-evnts-list-15-16.pdf (accessed 10 July 2018)

NHS England (2016) *Integrated Key Performance Indicators.* Leeds: NHS England. Available at: www.england.nhs.uk/publication/integrated-urgent-care-key-performance-indicators-201617/ (accessed 10 July 2018)

National Institute for Health and Care Excellence (2007) *CG50: Acutely Ill Patients in Hospital: recognition of and response to acute illness in adults in hospital.* London: NICE.

National Institute for Health and Care Excellence (2011) *CG123: Common Mental Health Problems: identification and pathways to care.* London: NICE.

National Institute for Health and Care Excellence (2015a) *NG9: Bronchiolitis in Children: diagnosis and management.* London: NICE.

National Institute for Health and Care Excellence (2015b) *NG31: Care of Dying Adults in the Last Days of Life.* London: NICE.

National Institute for Health and Care Excellence (2016) *NG61: End of Life Care for Infants, Children and Young People with Life-limiting Conditions: planning and management.* London: NICE.

National Institute for Health and Care Excellence (2017) *CG160: Fever in Under 5s: assessment and initial management.* London: NICE.

NMC and GMC (2015) *Openness and Honesty when Things go Wrong: the professional duty of candour.* London: Nursing and Midwifery Council and General Medical Council. Available at: www.nmc.org.uk/globalassets/sitedocuments/nmc-publications/openness-and-honesty-professional-duty-of-candour.pdf (last accessed 18 July 2018)

Nursing and Midwifery Council (2015) *The Code: standards of conduct, performance and ethics for nurses and midwives.* London: NMC. Available at: www.nmc.org.uk/globalassets/sitedocuments/nmc-publications/nmc-code.pdf (last accessed 10 July 2018)

Pope, B.B, Rodzen, L. and Spross, G. (2008) Raising the SBAR: how better communication improves patient outcomes. *Nursing,* 38(3): 41–43.

Purling, A. and King, L. (2012) A literature review: graduate nurses' preparedness for recognising and responding to the deteriorating patient. *Journal of Clinical Nursing,* 21(23–24): 3451–3465.

Royal College of Physicians (2012) *National Early Warning Score (NEWS) Standardising the assessment of acute-illness severity in the NHS.* London: RCP.

Royal College of Physicians (2017) *National Early Warning Score (NEWS2): standardising the assessment of acute-illness severity in the NHS.* London: RCP. Available at: www.rcplondon.ac.uk/projects/outputs/national-early-warning-score-news-2 (last accessed 18 July 2018)

Smith, G.B., Prytherch, D.R., Schmidt, P. *et al.* (2006) Hospital-wide physiological surveillance – a new approach to the early identification and management of the sick patient. *Resuscitation*, **71**(1): 19–28.

Subbe, C.P., Kruger, M., Rutherford, P. and Gemmel, L. (2001) Validation of a modified Early Warning Score in medical admissions. *Quarterly Journal of Medicine*, **94**(10): 521–526.

WHAT TO DO NEXT

1. Review local escalation procedures, tools, and complaints procedures when you start in practice.

2. Discuss with your preceptor potential challenging situations that may arise within your practice setting.

3. Identify key training required to demonstrate competent use of escalation charts, forms and equipment in the practice setting.

4. Ask senior nurses and/or your preceptor to observe you completing track and trigger charts and incident forms, to ensure you are competent.

5. Organise attendance at quality assurance, clinical governance or clinical incident review meetings, to increase your understanding of local quality improvement processes.

6. Establish whether conflict resolution and de-escalation training programmes are available to you when you start in practice.

7. Review local HR policies and guidelines relating to bullying and harassment and zero tolerance of aggression towards staff.

8. Review local policies relating to patient death and last offices.

CHAPTER 9

STRUCTURING YOUR FUTURE LEARNING AND SUPPORT

❝ *When you qualify you think 'great, no more lectures at university', but training and development is just beginning, it never ends – that's what makes nursing so interesting! It's important to have a support system around you throughout your career, not just at the beginning. I needed extra support at 12 months as I was delegated more, but I was still new and I wanted help going forward. I joined a band 5 support group which was really good. We could be honest and reflect on how difficult a shift was with our team leader who supported us. Managers asked us to feed back anything that would help us in our band 5 role. We asked for extra teaching on new treatments that were starting in our area, and got it.* ❞

18 months post-qualified nurse

❝ *I thought I'd automatically be offered funding to do a mentor course or a specialist course. I found out how funding for nurse education works and that budgets are set a year ahead. You need to plan your career to have the best chance of funding for courses and getting to a band 6. I had to have an interview as too many ward staff wanted to do the same course. I was given funding as I was a link nurse and showed how I would use the course to improve patient care.* ❞

2 years post-qualified children's nurse, promoted to band 6 specialist nurse

Many qualified nurses contact me at around 9–12 months post-qualification, for career advice or additional support in their band 5 role. Their requests usually relate to the following questions: "*Where can I access support to help develop my knowledge, skills or confidence as a band 5?"*, *"Where do I go from here?"*, *"How can I progress to a band 6?"* and *"How can I secure funding for a post-qualification course?"*. This chapter attempts to answer these important questions, offering guidance to plan your development and positively progress your career.

9.1 PROACTIVELY STRUCTURE YOUR LEARNING AND DEVELOPMENT

As a newly appointed staff nurse in a busy neurosurgical unit, I had a passion for nurse education but was unsure how to fulfil my aspirations. In 1993, my frustration resulted in a letter published in the *Nursing Times* entitled *'Informed help wanted on making post-basic education choices'*, calling for a *'career officer'* to advise nurses how to achieve their career aspirations (Kirrane, 1993). I meet many third year students and newly qualified nurses today who experience the same dilemma and are unsure how to navigate career structures and plan their future development.

During my early career, I had to direct my own development and self-fund academic courses, and there was a shortage of nursing posts to apply for. In contrast, today you have a multitude of posts to apply for, and access to national funding opportunities that may help progress your career.

Align your career to relevant skills and qualifications early on

UK health care employers are struggling to retain nurses and the promotion of structured career pathways, and of continuing professional development, is vital in order to retain our future nursing workforce (House of Commons Health Committee, 2018). Near the end of your first year qualified you will start to think about whether to continue as a band 5, or plan for a future band 6, and whether to remain in your chosen speciality or move to a new field (see *Box 3.3* in *Chapter 3* for example nursing roles/fields). Whichever pathway you choose, you need to start identifying the clinical skills and qualifications required to support lifelong learning.

The earlier you start to align professional and academic requirements to a career pathway, the more chance you have of successfully achieving your aspirations. Ask experienced staff for advice if you are unsure how to develop your career pathway. You may wish to rotate into different areas as a band 5 first, to experience different types of nursing and develop transferable skills. Not all nurses have ambitions to rise up the career ladder, and you may have no desire to become a band 6. This decision should be respected, as band 5s are the backbone of the health service, and essential to the delivery of direct patient care. However, band 5s still need to keep their clinical skills up to date through post-registration courses and study days applicable to their role.

Example career pathways for four key areas, *'Clinical'*, *'Education'*, *'Advanced practice'* and *'Research'*, are presented in *Table 9.1*. Each career pathway aligns nurse banding to example professional development and academic courses. Always check local job descriptions when applying for posts or deciding which career pathway is suitable. Employers will establish 'desirable' and 'essential' professional and academic requirements for individual jobs. The academic courses listed in *Table 9.1* are ideal, and some employers will not request this academic level prior to shortlisting for interviews.

On qualification, I always knew the area of nursing I wished to pursue was education. My career aspirations were aligned to professional qualifications and academic courses, using a similar framework to *Table 9.1*. To help identify the essential qualifications required, I initially checked with nurse tutors who advised me to commence a part-time BSc (Hons) degree in Nursing Studies at the Royal College of Nursing whilst working full-time. A postgraduate diploma in Education enabled me to register as a nurse tutor and helped my future promotion as a clinical development sister. Eventually I completed a Masters in advanced nursing practice, which supported my appointment as a lecturer practitioner (LP) 20 years ago, and this continues to be my ideal job. The key strategies I used to develop my early career still apply today.

Strategies to help you choose the right career pathway

Talk to staff working in the field

- Talk to staff working in the role that you wish to pursue, to increase your insights. Establish whether the role meets your expectations (the reality may be different to what you expected).
- Talk to senior staff (includes medics/AHPs) who understand your chosen career pathway, to get advice on progression.
- Establish a global picture of opportunities for career development across the service, through discussion with experienced staff.
- Review UK professional websites, such as the RCN, that present excellent online career resources.

Table 9.1: Example career pathways aligned to professional development and education

Nursing band and posts	Professional development	Academic course
Clinical post		
Band 5: staff nurse, community nurse, district nurse	NMC registered Interest shown in specialist area	BSc nursing degree
Band 6: senior staff nurse/deputy sister/charge nurse (CN), community nursing sister	NMC registered Experienced 1–2 years in specialist area Supervising and assessing in practice Active interest demonstrated in area e.g. *'link role'* or assisted band 7s Completed service project in the area	BSc nursing degree Post-qualification certificate in specialist area, e.g. oncology short course Postgraduate diploma in management/leadership/public health/finance
Band 7: sister/charge nurse, community team leader, community manager	NMC registered Experienced 2–3 years in specialist area Previously worked as band 6 Supervising and assessing in practice Leadership or project management experience Experience managing teams/others	BSc nursing degree Postgraduate certificate in specialist area or management/leadership Postgraduate diploma Masters relating to health care, leadership, management, public health or finance
Band 8/9: matron/divisional nurse, community matron, senior commissioning manager	NMC registered Experienced 4–5 years in health care (not necessarily the specialist area) Supervising and assessing in practice Experience as a band 7 delivering and leading nursing teams Demonstrates leadership, management or project management experience Experience of financial management or writing business plans	Postgraduate diploma in leadership, finance or project management Masters relating to advanced nursing practice, health care, leadership, management, public health or finance

Table 9.1: *(Continued)*

Nursing band and posts	Professional development	Academic course
Educational post		
Band 5: staff nurse, community nurse, district nurse	NMC registered Interest shown in education	BSc nursing degree
Band 6: practice development nurse, clinical nurse educator, clinical educator, community training nurse	NMC registered Experienced 1–2 years in health care Supervising and assessing in practice Active interest demonstrated in education, e.g. *'educator link role'*, delivered teaching or written educational documents, such as competencies	BSc nursing degree Post-qualification certificate in education Postgraduate certificate in education
Band 7: practice development education lead, corporate educator, education facilitator, care home education lead, Macmillan facilitator and practice educator	NMC registered Experienced 2–3 years in health care Previously worked in a band 6 education role (an education role may link to transferable skills, e.g. a team leader may demonstrate teaching within a team) Supervising and assessing in practice Leadership or project management experience Experience managing others	BSc nursing degree Postgraduate certificate in education Postgraduate diploma, ideally Masters relating to health care, leadership, education or management
Band 8/9: corporate / trust divisional education lead / lecturer practitioner, senior public health educator	NMC registered Experienced 4–5 years in health care field Supervising and assessing in practice Experience planning and delivering educational programmes	Health related (Hons) degree (post holder could be a nurse or other AHP) Corporate / trust divisional education lead should have Masters relating to health care leadership, education or management

(continued)

Table 9.1: (Continued)

Nursing band and posts	Professional development	Academic course
	Leadership, management or project management experience Experience managing teams Experience of financial management and writing business plans	Lecturer practitioner should have Masters in education, advanced practice or health care; usually working towards, or having completed, a doctorate/PhD

Specialist/advanced nursing practice post

Nursing band and posts	Professional development	Academic course
Band 5: staff nurse, community nurse, district nurse	NMC registered Interest shown in specialist area	BSc nursing degree
Band 6: specialist nurse/specialist practitioner/clinical governance nurse, community practitioner, community public health nurse	NMC registered Experienced 1 year in specialist field Supervising and assessing in practice Active interest demonstrated in specialist area, e.g. *'link role'* in the area or related service improvement/research project	BSc nursing degree Post-qualification certificate in specialist area Accredited nurse prescribing qualification or course Postgraduate diploma in advanced nursing practice or autonomous health care practice
Band 7: advanced nurse practitioner, community advanced practitioner, integrated urgent care advanced practitioner, community health practitioner	NMC registered Experienced 2–3 years in specialist field Previously worked in a band 6 role Supervising and assessing in practice Leadership or project management experience Experience managing others	BSc nursing degree Post-qualification certificate in specialist area Accredited nurse prescribing qualification or course Postgraduate diploma Masters in autonomous health care practice or advanced nursing practice
Band 8/9: service manager to senior advanced nurse practitioners/nurse consultant, community advanced practitioner service manager	NMC registered Experienced 4–5 years in health care field Preferable to have experience in specialist area (not always essential if transferable skills can be shown)	BSc nursing degree Accredited qualification in management, leadership or project management

Table 9.1: (Continued)

Nursing band and posts	Professional development	Academic course
	Supervising and assessing in practice Project management experience Leadership and managerial experience Experience managing teams Experience of financial management	Masters in autonomous health care practice or advanced nursing practice Nurse consultant should have Masters and doctorate/PhD (or working towards doctorate)

Research post

Nursing band and posts	Professional development	Academic course
Band 5: research nurse, public health nurse	NMC registered Interest shown in research or specialist area	BSc (Hons) nursing degree
Band 6: clinical research nurse, clinical trials nurse researcher, community researcher	NMC registered Experienced 1 year in health care field Supervising and assessing in practice Experience in specialist area, e.g. endocrinology if diabetes research post Active interest demonstrated in research area, e.g. link nurse role or research project	BSc (Hons) nursing degree Research course/qualification Post-qualification certificate or diploma in specialist area
Band 7: clinical research practitioner, research project manager, trials project manager, community research practitioner	NMC/AHP-registered qualification Experienced 2–3 years in health care field Supervising and assessing in practice Previously worked in a band 6 role Research and project management experience Leadership experience Experience managing others	Health-related (Hons) degree (could be nurse or other AHP) Research module/course Post-qualification certificate or diploma in specialist area Project management or leadership qualification Postgraduate diploma Masters that is health related

(continued)

Table 9.1: (Continued)

Nursing band and posts	Professional development	Academic course
Band 8: clinical research operational manager / research team service manager	NMC / AHP registered qualification Experienced 4–5 years in health care field Supervising and assessing in practice Previously worked in a band 7 role Preferable to have experience in specialist area but not always essential Project management experience Leadership and managerial experience Experience managing teams Experience of financial management	Health-related (Hons) degree (post holder could be a nurse or other AHP) Research qualification Project management qualification Masters in leadership, management or finance Working towards doctorate / PhD

Observe staff at work

- Arrange an informal visit and observe staff at work.
- Use visits as opportunities to network with others and demonstrate your interest in the area. Staff may offer additional time in the field, e.g. attending clinics or patient groups.

Attend progress reviews and appraisals

- Discuss which career pathway is best suited to your skill set during progression review meetings, which inform your future development plans.
- Ask your line manager to support your career progression and attendance on related study days / courses.
- Arrange an annual appraisal to discuss your current role and to set your objectives, individualised development plans and/or SMART goals.

Achieve the level of qualification, experience and clinical skills required

- Review local job descriptions and personal specifications to establish the *'essential'* and *'desirable'* experience, skills and qualifications required for the role.

- Review relevant band 6/7 job descriptions in the area (you can request job descriptions from your local HR department or view national examples online at www.jobs.nhs.uk).
- Align your future practice and development towards achieving the required qualification, experience and clinical skills.
- If another setting offers you more chance of courses or relevant experience, you may need to consider a move.

Show passion and enthusiasm

- Show passion and enthusiasm for your specialist area:
  - act as a band 5 link nurse
  - attend local and national study days/conferences in the field
  - use media tools/online forums to keep up to date with local and national developments
  - complete a project that links to the role, e.g. a specialist care plan.

Share your aspirations

- Share your goals and aspirations with your manager or those in the field (if they know you are interested in pursuing a goal they are more likely to offer potential opportunities).

Show resilience

- Never give up on pursuing your goals because someone says you are not *'ready'*. Listen to feedback from your manager/preceptor as you may not have the required skills yet. If you do not agree, you can ask an independent senior nurse or educator what they think too.
- Successful people learn to become resilient and will keep aspiring to reach their goals through adversity *(I went for two team leader posts before I was appointed following my third interview!)*.

9.2 WHAT YOU SHOULD EXPECT OVER THE NEXT YEAR AND ONWARDS

In 2012, an extensive review of UK nurse education by the Willis Commission examined support and education for newly registered nurses. Recommendations urged nursing employers to *'recognise, fund, promote and support nurses' continuing professional development'*, as an investment for the future (Willis, 2012). Newly qualified UK doctors benefit from a national mandatory clinical training programme for 2 years. The package consists of regular supervisory sessions and an online system of monitoring progression (Academy of Medical Royal Colleges, 2016). In comparison, there are no national regulations or minimum criteria set during your first 2 years qualified as a nurse.

Throughout your career you are continually required to write annual objectives/goals, following an appraisal review with your line manager. To help structure your learning, an example year-long pathway for professional development reviews (PDRs) is presented in *Chapter 2*, along with example objectives and tips to write SMART goals.

Following your preceptorship period, ongoing professional development, training and support will continue, as determined by your employer and according to local guidelines and policies. It is important to identify the local structures employed to organise your PDRs to support your future training and development needs. Although your preceptor is responsible for offering individual support over your preceptorship period and onwards, it is your responsibility to direct your own professional development throughout your career. An example of what is expected during your preceptorship year and afterwards is presented in *Table 9.2*.

Annual appraisal

An appraisal is the act of making a judgement on somebody or something. Health care regulators such as the CQC and Department of Health advocate that all health care employers should provide an annual appraisal for their staff, as it is deemed essential to promoting high quality care (DH, 2004; Department of Health, Social Services and Public Safety, 2015). Annual NHS staff surveys and health service reviews regularly measure the percentage of staff *'compliant with annual appraisals'* to indicate the quality of staff support within an area. The higher the percentage of staff completing an appraisal on time, the greater the level of compliance and quality of staff support indicated.

Many NHS employers have an online RED, AMBER and GREEN system to highlight when appraisals are due. Staff due an appraisal in the next month are highlighted on the system as AMBER; staff past their annual appraisal date are highlighted in RED, and staff meeting their date will be GREEN. The system simultaneously alerts the person who is due an appraisal and their line manager, to give them both an incentive to complete the appraisal.

Table 9.2: What is expected during your preceptorship year and onwards

Key area	Details
Professional development reviews (PDRs)	Usually 3–6-monthly over the preceptorship period PDRs continue annually for the rest of your career but can be requested more frequently
Training packages and programmes	E-learning packages and statutory and mandatory training continue to require updating throughout your career Training updates are annual or 2–3-yearly (local policy and educators will confirm timelines)
Band 5 core and specialist competencies	Some employers offer band 5 and 6 competencies to help develop staff competence and leadership and management skills Experienced band 5s are expected to start assisting band 6s in aspects of their role, especially if working towards a band 6 (*it is helpful to review band 6 job descriptions/competencies to establish what you are working towards*)
Post-qualification specialist training/courses	There are local and national specialist study days, workbooks and/or courses relating to a band 5 role and aspirations Your preceptor and local educator will advise you on appropriate training and educational courses
Annual appraisal	Appraisals are linked to previous PDRs and structured according to frameworks, such as the NHS Knowledge and Skills Framework (NHS KSF) (DH, 2004); themes from the NMC *Code* (2015a); and local job description/competencies or employer priorities (see the appraisal pointers in *Box 9.1*)
3-yearly NMC revalidation	NMC (2018b) revalidation is linked to your PDR/appraisal and a personal portfolio containing your revalidation reflections and practice-related feedback (see the revalidation pointers in *Table 9.3*)
Supervision and assessment	When confident and competent as a band 5, you will be expected to supervise and assess nursing assistants, students or newly qualified nurses (see section on acting as a practice supervisor and practice assessor, below)

What is covered in my appraisal?

During an annual appraisal, your progress throughout the year should be constructively assessed and evaluated by your line manager. An annual appraisal usually covers:

- how your role relates to the rest of the team/organisation
- personal and professional development over the last year
- your current knowledge and skills in line with requirements for the role
- your achievements using previously set role-specific objectives and/or SMART goals
- your current competence/performance using a job description and/or competencies
- education and training opportunities available to you over the next year
- additional support to access over the next year if required
- future career progression and/or options to develop within your current role
- future objectives and priorities which are set as part of your personal development plan.

How is an appraisal structured?

As part of your ongoing development, you should be offered an annual appraisal by your line manager for the rest of your career. Your preceptor may or may not be your line manager, and it is important that you find out who your line manager is and who is responsible for conducting your appraisal. Your first appraisal should take place at the end of year one post-qualification, during which you will set goals and objectives for the next year post-qualification. Appraisals and related documentation should remain confidential at all times and be conducted in a closed, private room.

The person conducting your appraisal is called an **appraiser** and you are the **appraisee**.

There is no national system or structure for nursing appraisals and UK employers use a variety of frameworks and headings on appraisal documentation, such as:

- **NHS Knowledge and Skills Framework (KSF) (DH, 2004):**
  - communication
  - personal and people development
  - health, safety and security
  - service improvement
  - quality
  - equality and diversity.

- NMC *Code* (NMC, 2015a) themes:
  - prioritise people
  - practise effectively
  - preserve safety
  - promote professionalism and trust.
- Band 5 competency frameworks or job descriptors
- **Other local frameworks or structures:** aligned to employer mission statements or trust strategy/quality priorities, such as *'compassionate care and respect'*.

Aim to become familiar with appraisal frameworks within your local area, which may be paper-based or online. Within my local trust PDRs, annual appraisals and NMC portfolios for revalidation are set up for each nurse using an integrated online system. The system enables nurses to link past PDR reviews and reflections to their three-yearly NMC revalidation meeting with their line manager.

The need for constructive communication

Once you secure a date for an annual appraisal, you should prepare well in advance to gain the best out of your appraisal. *'Your'* is the operative word here, as an appraisal is a chance for you to receive constructive feedback and support from your manager to enable you to become the best you can in your role. Some guidance to inform your future appraisals is presented in *Box 9.1.*

Box 9.1 Guidance and tips to support your appraisal

Preparation before appraisal

Be proactive

- Proactively book your appraisal well in advance of your due date, as managers deal with fluctuating workloads that can lead to cancelled appraisals. Check with your appraiser how they prefer you to book, e.g. by email, verbally or via calendar invitation through an administrator.

Don't worry

- There is no need to worry before your appraisal, as your line manager should lead you through local structures. Appraisal frameworks tend to be user-friendly as they need to fit with all staff needs.

Familiarise yourself with the appraisal template

- Review your appraisal template before your meeting. Usually under each headed section on an appraisal template there will be two spaces/comment boxes, one for you and one for your appraiser, to write/type the following in some form:
    1. How you have progressed relating to your job descriptors or previous objectives/SMART goals
    2. How your current role relates to your team/the organisation
    3. What has been achieved by you since the last appraisal (personally and professionally)
    4. What additional support or training opportunities will help you progress in the future
    5. What your objectives/development plans are for the next year

Find out what your line manager expects you to prepare

- Prior to your appraisal, write notes on the areas 1–5 above to bring with you, or actual evidence of achievement, e.g. within a professional portfolio.
- Some appraisers are happy to chat through progression with limited preparation on your part. Others will request evidence of achievement, e.g. signed competencies. Prior to your appraisal, check what measures your appraiser will use to evaluate your progression.

During appraisal

Make your own notes

- It is easy to forget what has been discussed in an appraisal. You can make your own notes during your appraisal and/or complete an online appraisal template as you go along with your appraiser.
- I tend to type up summary notes as each appraisal section is reviewed with the staff member present; this ensures that we both agree with the content.
- Some staff prefer to write final notes in more neatly later when they have more time to reflect on the meeting.

Consider your performance

- Your appraiser will review your personal qualities, knowledge, competence and skills using key measures, such as band 5 competencies, job descriptions, personal specifications, learning objectives and SMART goals.

- Consider your own performance and achievements over the previous year using related measures to summarise your progression.

Communication should be two-way and constructive

- Two-way communication is an essential part of an appraisal. You should have the opportunity to give your perspective when discussing your performance and discuss areas where you require extra support.
- You may not achieve previously set objectives/goals, due to a lack of opportunity or support. An appraisal is an appropriate forum for you to discuss reasons for any lack of achievement that will assist your line manager to plan additional future support.

Use constructive feedback to inform your future practice

- Managers should be trained to appraise staff and give constructive feedback on staff performance over the year. You, in turn, need to listen and receive constructive feedback from an experienced nurse, to develop your future knowledge, skills and competence.
- If you do not agree with your appraisal feedback, then constructively state why. Offer your appraiser factual examples to demonstrate your points and support your different perspective.

Acknowledge personal issues that impact on performance

- We all have lives outside of work and sometimes personal/social issues may impact on our ability to function at work, such as a divorce, bereavement or ill health. Most managers are experienced at supporting staff through difficult times. If you are struggling, you may wish to discuss personal issues as part of your appraisal. You do not have to share aspects of your home life if it makes you uncomfortable and you can access additional support services yourself.

Summary and future plans

Align your career aspirations

- When asking your manager to consider you for a future promotion, or specialist courses, do your homework and identify exactly what you need in order to achieve your aspirations.
- Some employers will not even consider requests for a future course without the course being formally requested and documented in the staff member's appraisal.

Setting objectives and personal development plans for the next year

- Following your appraisal, new objectives and/or SMART goals are set for completion over the next year. Your line manager / local educators can help you write these if you need extra support.
- Personal development plans will need to be updated with new review dates.
- Opportunities for additional training and support should be included in the above plans.

Complete paperwork

- Once all relevant sections within your appraisal template are complete, your appraisal can be signed off by both you and your appraiser.
- Signing off your appraisal indicates that you have both read the content and reviewed the other person's views.
- If using an online system make sure it states *'Completed'* or turns GREEN on the system, as it is easy to forget to follow through the online signatures. You may need to prompt your manager to complete their side of the sign-off.
- Never sign off your appraisal without stating your view in the comments section. If you are unhappy with the comments made by your appraiser then voice this in your appraisal; ensure your perspective is documented, and that you receive a copy of the completed appraisal for your own records.
- You can request further advice from your HR department if needed.

Make a diary / calendar note for your next appraisal

What happens if I am not progressing as expected?

If a member of staff informs you that you are not progressing well, they should do this in a supportive, constructive and professional manner, i.e. not at the bedside in earshot of patients! You need to consider the ability of the person voicing concerns, as there is a big difference between a disgruntled nursing assistant who has worked with you once, compared with a team leader who has worked closely with you for the last year.

If a senior nurse informs you that you are not meeting expectations, they should be explicit as to what you need to improve on, and how they will support you to achieve a positive outcome. If you are deemed by your line manager to be underperforming in your role, they should deal with performance issues outside of an appraisal, according to local procedure. Examples of these include *'managing work performance procedure'* or *'disciplinary procedure'*. It is inappropriate to be line managed as part of an appraisal, and the management of staff performance should initially focus on supporting the employee to help them improve their performance to meet the standard required.

During a preceptorship period it is acknowledged that newly qualified staff may require additional supervision and support. Unless there is evidence of serious or gross misconduct, a lack of progression as a band 5 is usually dealt with **informally** at first; however, actions must adhere to local procedure. Even during an informal phase, it is important that you review local procedures to ensure you receive adequate support from your manager to improve the area(s) of concern.

Most nursing contracts include a **3–6-month probationary period** that provides a safety net for employers after they have recruited you. The probationary period is a period of time where your ability to perform at the required level is observed and assessed. If you fail to achieve the standard within the probationary period, your employer can dismiss you without concerns of unfair dismissal and employment tribunals later. If you are unsure of procedures, or concerned about the way you are being supported, talk to your local HR department.

During an **informal stage** you should be offered the following:

- **An initial meeting with your manager** where your manager should:
  - state what they expect from you
  - detail the specific area(s) of your practice that you need to improve upon
  - provide details of how progress will be measured, e.g. competency achievement
  - propose a future plan of support to help improve your performance
  - give you an opportunity to discuss your perspective of the situation
  - provide a copy of documentation from the meeting for your records.
- **A performance improvement plan (PIP)** should be written that clearly sets out the area of concern; objectives and/or SMART goals to be achieved; how success (the outcome) will be measured; along with timescales.

- **Future progress review meetings** – you should be made aware of future progress review meetings in advance, along with information on who is attending and reviewing your progress. An example of this might be a weekly progress review meeting with your ward sister present and a practice development nurse to assess band 5 competency achievement. Often managers will oversee a PIP and lead a review meeting, but will expect a team leader or clinical educator to sign off SMART goals or band 5 competencies.

- **Documentation** – you should receive a copy of your PIP documentation; review meetings and any related objectives; competencies/SMART goals, for the duration. There should be space on review documentation for you to write your perspective of the situation, e.g. whether you are happy/unhappy with support offered, or find any aspects of the process difficult. Additionally, you may be required to write reflections or include self-assessments as part of the PIP. The documentation you receive should accurately and factually detail what was covered in meetings. Although you are not being formally performance managed at this stage, records from an informal discussion can remain on a person's file for 6 months.

- **Additional support/training** – your individual learning needs should be reviewed and additional support offered to help you achieve set objectives/goals, e.g. specialist training days or additional clinical educator support at the bedside.

The majority of nurses who complete a PIP go on to have fulfilling careers with no further performance issues. However, you should be aware that if you are assessed as not improving with additional PIP support, your employer could move to a formal disciplinary stage. Local procedures usually contain a flow chart that includes the following stages:

- **Informal meeting**
- **PIP review meetings**
- **First formal meeting** (potential written warning)
- **Second formal meeting** (potential final written warning)
- **Formal performance hearing** (potential dismissal)
- **Appeals meeting.**

(*Always check the details of local procedures: 'Managing work performance procedure' or 'Disciplinary procedure'.*)

Following any formal action, it is important that you take independent legal advice, which is covered by your union subscriptions. **NOTE: never work in practice without union cover as this provides full indemnity cover and legal advice/representation when you need it.**

Following cases of gross misconduct, such as violence towards a patient, an employee can be dismissed with immediate effect and without notice or payment.

The importance of NMC registration and revalidation

When you complete your degree, you will be directed by the university programme lead to complete paperwork applying for your first NMC registration, as a registered nurse (RN) or registered midwife (RM). You are required to pay annual NMC fees to register and receive a personal NMC PIN number. Your first employer will request evidence of an active NMC PIN number before you sign a formal employment contract, which means you must register with the NMC prior to starting your first post.

Throughout the rest of your career you are required to:

- **pay an annual NMC fee to remain on the NMC register**
- **complete an NMC online process called revalidation every 3 years to maintain your NMC registration.**

It is your responsibility to pay annual registration fees and revalidate every 3 years before NMC expiry dates. To ensure that your registration does not lapse, you must register with NMC Online and actively check that fee payments go through on time. Your NMC registration will lapse and your NMC account will be deemed inactive if fees are not paid or you do not complete your revalidation on time.

It is illegal to work as an RN or RM (in any circumstances) if you are unregistered. NMC Online sends you a reminder when fees are due or your registration is near to lapsing (currently sent 60 days before expiry or revalidation date). It is important to inform the NMC of any changes to your home/email addresses to receive these vital reminders.

What happens if my NMC registration lapses by accident?

Reputable health care employers will not accept reasons for lapses in NMC registration, as you are essentially working illegally as an RN/RM. I have heard excuses such as '*I was on annual/maternity leave*', '*I didn't receive an NMC warning as my computer had a virus*', '*I moved house*' or '*I didn't have enough money in the bank*', none of which is recognised as a valid reason. You are accountable and responsible for registering with NMC Online and can view your account to ascertain fees and revalidation expiry dates. If you allow your NMC registration to expire, your employer will usually stop payment of your wages (including maternity/sick pay) for all unregistered days, which includes any days off. All of which gives you a good incentive to keep in date!

If you suddenly realise that your NMC registration has expired and you are at work, you must stop working immediately and inform your line manager that you have identified a lapsed registration. This is dealt with formally and line managers will request that you leave the clinical setting immediately. Employers usually start a disciplinary procedure as your absence can affect staffing, it will impact on service provision and your insurance at work is invalid without registration. You will be called to a first formal warning meeting and receive a first formal letter from your employer, which must be highlighted on future references. Following a lapse in registration, it can take between 2 and 6 weeks to rectify through the NMC. If you are found to be working unregistered your application may be referred to the NMC Registrar's Advisory Group. In summary, don't ever let your NMC registration lapse!

How do I revalidate every three years?

Since April 2016, an NMC revalidation process must be followed by all RNs/RMs every 3 years to maintain their NMC registration (NMC, 2018b). If it is your first time revalidating, do not worry as most employers are used to the process. A few tips are presented below:

- Ensure that your revalidation is completed by **the first day of the month in which your registration expires.**

- The revalidation process requires someone to act as a '*Confirmer*', usually your line manager, to verify that you have the required number of practice hours and evidence of continuous practice development (see *Table 9.3*). It is helpful to identify who your NMC confirmer is, so you can chat through the process.

- Plan your revalidation review well in advance as managers can be busy (as early as 6 months before your revalidation due date).

- Prepare your revalidation evidence prior to the meeting to make the process as easy as possible for your confirmer.

Table 9.3: NMC requirements for revalidation every 3 years (NMC, 2018b)

NMC requirements	Evidence and examples
Practice hours over the last 3 years	**A minimum of 450 hours** if already registered with NMC (**900 hours** if renewing registration). Usually your manager will have access to e-rosters that demonstrate your practice hours. If not, you must provide information on shifts worked, e.g. employment contract, timesheets.
Continuous practice development (CPD)	**35 hours of CPD (20 hours of which must be participatory learning)** Participatory learning includes any learning activity where you interact with other people, e.g. study group, conference or group forum on a virtual environment. You must demonstrate accurate records of your CPD recorded in hours and the types of development, e.g. records on your e-learning account; band 5 competencies achieved in practice; certificates from completed academic and professional courses, study days or course workbooks. You must demonstrate how you have related your CPD to practice, which can be verbally discussed or written notes – NMC (2018b) templates are helpful. **Do not include personal data** on revalidation documents.
Practice-related feedback	**Five accounts of practice-related feedback** A range of practice-related feedback can be used, such as patients' thank you cards; feedback from colleagues; evaluations from student nurses that you have supervised; evaluations from teaching.
Reflective accounts	**Five written reflective accounts** You will be used to providing reflection and should use a familiar reflective tool. Reflective accounts should demonstrate what you have learnt and how this has influenced your practice. You may reflect on situations that went well or you might learn from a difficult situation. A simple reflection linked to an element of patient care or your practice is ideal. Reflective accounts can align to your CPD activity, practice-related feedback or any other event or experience.
A reflective discussion	**An NMC reflective discussion** A reflective discussion summary must be completed using correct NMC forms (NMC, 2018b) and stored as paper copy.

(continued)

Table 9.3: (Continued)

NMC requirements	Evidence and examples
	The reflective discussion record includes: • name and NMC PIN of the NMC-registered RN / RM that you had the discussion with • date you had the discussion. If your line manager is not NMC registered, you must discuss your reflective accounts with another NMC-registered person.
Health and character	Making a health and character declaration is completed as part of your online application.
Professional indemnity	Appropriate indemnity arrangements must be in place, e.g. through a professional body (RCN), Unison or a private insurance arrangement.

• Ensure that you review current NMC revalidation processes, forms, templates and resources prior to your revalidation as they are very helpful (NMC, 2018b).

• You must register with NMC Online to complete your revalidation form, which verifies you have met with your confirmer and have met the criteria required to revalidate.

Creating a professional portfolio

An up-to-date and well-organised professional portfolio will provide clear evidence of your skills, development and practice experiences. A good portfolio can inform future PDRs and provide evidence for a 3-yearly revalidation review (as long as practice-related feedback and reflective accounts are up to date). Portfolios can also support future job applications or requests for educational funding.

A portfolio is a personal reflection of you as a person, as well as a record of your progression. You can be creative when presenting your evidence, as long as it is organised clearly and covers the key elements required. As a younger generation of tech-savvy students are qualifying, I am reviewing portfolios that are imaginatively presented using visuals, audio files or electronic formats. Staff who suffer from a disability can use a variety of ways to personalise the format of their portfolio to suit their learning needs. Similarly, when discussing your revalidation with your confirmer they should be flexible with the format used to demonstrate evidence. I recently attended a revalidation where the person had recorded a series of verbal reflections using audio files, rather than writing them, due to his dyslexia. Whichever method you use, the same rules apply relating to data protection and confidentiality. Most professional portfolios I review are paper-based or electronic e-portfolios. There are excellent example portfolio templates relating to both methods from the RCN (2018) and NMC (2018b). A hard copy portfolio may become obsolete, but many interviewees print out an e-portfolio for the interviewer to review during interviews.

If you wish to design your own portfolio structure, there is no specific order when you are dividing sections. I have read portfolios starting with a patient thank you card, for example, or one quote from practice-related feedback, to introduce themselves as a compassionate person. Structuring your portfolio really depends on your contents and how they relate to each section. You should always present evidence clearly using defined sections to make it flow easily for the reader and demonstrate good organisation. Your portfolio will usually contain a number of headed sections; see examples and helpful pointers in *Table 9.4*.

Table 9.4: Your professional portfolio

Section	Pointers
Title and contents	**Clearly signpost:** signpost your portfolio content using a contents page or a list of defined sections / headings. Paper-based portfolios can be placed in a folder using plastic wallets and dividing tabs. E-portfolio templates from the RCN (2018) and NMC (2018b) are already structured and you just need to upload evidence, e.g. electronic certificates following completion of e-learning packages.
Introduction	**Brief introduction:** your introduction should explain the purpose of the portfolio, your current role and the format used.
	Personal statement: include a brief personal statement at the start of your portfolio (or end) that provides a summary of your professional values, passions and career aspirations / goals. Your personal statement should briefly summarise previous experience. Example personal statements can be found in the RCN's (2018) *'Careers Resources for Nurses and Midwives'* to help guide you.
	Visual / oral introduction: creative portfolios use pictures, visual aids or audio files to introduce values and goals. You still need to provide context to your visual content to ensure the reader understands what you are trying to portray.

(continued)

Table 9.4: (Continued)

Section	Pointers
Current job description	**Band 5 job descriptions:** a copy of a band 5 job description will present your current responsibilities. Non-UK trained nurses working in the UK find this particularly helpful if they return home to explain a band 5/6 role, as career structures and responsibilities can differ across the globe.
Curriculum vitae (CV)	**CV format:** often a standard CV is used to introduce portfolios, as it contains details of education, employment and career aspirations, as well as personal interests. Remember to update your CV as you progress, especially when taking your portfolio to an interview. The RCN's (2018) *'Careers Resources for Nurses and Midwives'* provides excellent advice and example CVs to help you.
Continuous practice development (CPD)	See *Table 9.3* for example content and pointers.
Practice-related feedback	See *Table 9.3.*
Reflective accounts	See *Table 9.3.*
Achievements	**Professional and personal achievements:** aim to distinguish yourself above other candidates in this section by portraying your passion and motivation. Do not place a whole project in your portfolio; a summary or abstract will suffice. Include additional notes which can briefly explain how your achievements have influenced practice. Examples for this section include: • summary of project work or example work such as updated care plan or patient information leaflet • summary/abstract of service improvement project or research • PowerPoint from a teaching session • awards, scholarships and research bursaries • photos/narrative from recent events, e.g. employer newsletters • charity work/projects or interests that demonstrate transferable skills • publications – include hard copies of any journal publications.

Key tip: during your first few months qualified, start your professional portfolio and begin collecting evidence. Once your portfolio is structured, you can keep updating the evidence as you progress. Using a portfolio will assist future PDRs and revalidations, as you can more easily identify evidence for the reviewer (reviewers will be pleased, as a portfolio makes the process much easier!).

Acting as a practice supervisor and practice assessor

As a qualified nurse, you are expected to supervise and assess student nurses and nursing assistants in practice. Supervising, assessing and supporting junior colleagues is written into job descriptions as a band 5 responsibility. After anywhere between 6 and 18 months in your role, you may be asked to act as a practice supervisor for a student in practice. You can check with your line manager as to when they expect you to start supervising others and the types of assessments and competency frameworks they expect you to use. Practice supervisors are expected to contribute to a student's record of achievement by *'periodically recording relevant observations'* on students' conduct and proficiency (NMC, 2018a). They are expected *'to appropriately raise and respond to student conduct and competence concerns'* and engage with practice assessors to share relevant observations informing the achievement of proficiencies.

The new NMC (2018a) *'Standards for Education and Training Part 2: standards for student supervision and assessment'* require all registered nursing students to also be supported by a practice assessor (a more experienced nursing assessor) to confirm achievement of registered nurses' proficiencies and programme outcomes for practice learning. The practice assessor works in partnership with a nominated academic assessor to evaluate and recommend the student for progression for each part of their training programme.

The student practice supervisory and assessor roles being introduced by the NMC (2018a) are shown below, together with their responsibilities.

Academic assessors:

- collate and confirm student achievement of proficiencies and programme outcomes in the academic environment for each part of the programme
- record objective, evidence-based decisions on conduct, proficiency and achievement
- provide recommendations for progression, drawing on student records and other resources
- maintain current knowledge and expertise relevant for the proficiencies and programme outcomes they are assessing and confirming

- work in partnership with a nominated **practice assessor** to evaluate and recommend the student for progression for each part of their programme
- have an understanding of the student's learning and achievement in practice
- communicate and collaborate between **academic** and **practice assessors** at scheduled relevant points during student progression
- are not simultaneously the **practice supervisor** and **practice assessor** for the same student.

Practice assessors:

- **conduct assessments to confirm study achievement of proficiencies and programme outcomes for practice learning**
- make decisions informed by feedback received from **practice supervisors**
- make and record objective, evidence-based assessments on conduct, proficiency and achievement, drawing on student records and direct observation and student self-reflection
- maintain current knowledge and expertise relevant for the proficiencies and programme outcomes they are assessing
- work in partnership with a nominated **academic assessor** to evaluate and recommend the student for progression for each part of their programme
- have an understanding of the student's learning and achievement in theory
- communicate and collaborate between **practice** and **academic assessors** at scheduled relevant points during student progression
- are not simultaneously the **practice supervisor** and **academic assessor** for the same student
- undertake preparation or evidence prior learning experience that enables them to demonstrate:
  - interpersonal skills relevant to student learning and assessment
  - objective, evidence-based assessments of students
  - constructive feedback to facilitate professional development in others
  - knowledge of the assessment process and their role within it
- receive ongoing support and training to develop their role

- proactively develop their professional practice and knowledge to fulfil their role
- understand the proficiencies and programme outcomes that the students are aiming to achieve.

Practice supervisors:

- **contribute to the student's record of achievement by periodically recording relevant observations on the conduct, proficiency and achievement of the students they are supervising**
- contribute to student assessments to inform decisions for progression
- engage with **practice assessors** and **academic assessors** to share relevant observations on the conduct, proficiency and achievement of the students they are supervising
- appropriately raise and respond to student conduct and competence concerns
- receive ongoing support to prepare, reflect and develop effective supervisions and contribute to student learning and assessment
- understand the proficiencies and programme outcomes they are supporting students to achieve
- serve as role models for safe and effective practice in line with the Code of Conduct
- support and supervise students, providing feedback on their progress
- have current knowledge and experience in the area in which they are providing support and supervision
- receive ongoing support to participate in the practice learning of students.

Promoting personal resilience and accessing support

Bright (1997) was the first to observe that nurses spent an inordinate amount of time caring for others and should use a *'self-care approach'* towards their own support to develop *'personal resilience'*. To thrive as a qualified nurse, you need to devise strategies to respond to workload stresses, and build personal resilience to prevent burnout (Jackson *et al.*, 2007).

Throughout your training, you have been made aware of the need to monitor your stress levels at work, look out for signs of stress, and identify strategies to successfully manage and prevent stress. When you start in practice you are entitled to a preceptorship period of support, regular PDRs and annual appraisals. However, during your first year qualified you may still experience a sudden reality shock in practice, as you do not have a practice supervisor to immediately call upon to support your decisions. During your transition preceptorship period, you are at risk of reacting to pressures in busy health care environments, rather than proactively managing and looking after yourself.

When you start in practice, it is important to find out where you can access additional support to decrease your stress levels, achieve a good work/life balance, strengthen your resilience and maintain positivity at work. When advising new starters with their initial SMART goals, I always suggest three related actions to enable them to achieve this:

1. **Identify what is on offer locally and nationally that you can access for support.**

2. **Identify experienced colleague(s) in your practice area who are good role models that you can trust to confidentially share any concerns/anxieties and 'offload' to.**

3. **Proactively plan a supportive network around you:** there are many ways for nurses to access support, including one-to-one or group support, and different modes of delivery including face to face, online group forums and group meetings (see *Table 9.5* for more details).

Types of post-qualification courses

After a year qualified, you will probably start looking into what post-qualification courses are suitable for your future development, how to apply for them and who pays. Professional training within a specialist area does not always require a university level course. It is helpful to align your future career goals to academic courses, to establish which courses will best support your development (see *Section 9.1*).

University courses and the credit system

Higher education programmes, such as a BSc (Hons) degree or an MSc (Masters) are composed of a number of individual modules or units. When reviewing the types of university courses and modules available, there are different levels and credits to navigate. Most UK universities use the Quality Assurance Agency for Higher Education (QAA) (2009) credit system (see *Table 9.6*).

Table 9.5: Band 5 support available

Support	Pointers
One-to-one support	It is helpful to identify colleagues to confidentially share your anxieties and concerns with. You should access 1:1 support from experienced nurses or peers.
	Identify colleagues / peers who offer sound and professional advice. There is no point offloading to someone who is unsympathetic or just tells you to leave nursing. A good role model and advocate for nursing will realistically acknowledge your concerns, whilst constructively advising strategies to inform your future practice / learning.
	Contact your clinical education team or past university tutors for advice.
Local band 5 forum	Many employers offer group support to newly qualified staff that takes the form of band 5 forums.
	Band 5 forums may be offered in your local area or across numerous settings.
	Group forums are usually run by a senior nurse who facilitates discussions and offers supportive strategies.
	Topics for meetings are usually led according to the needs of the band 5s.
	Always take the opportunity to meet with your peers in group forums if offered; such groups can promote reassurance, as group members relate to each other's issues.
Team meeting or awayday	Team meetings and team awaydays involve a team (trained and untrained staff) spending time together to discuss how to solve team / practice issues and support each other.
	A manager / team leader usually leads the day using a planned agenda.
	Team awaydays usually occur once a year as they need planning around staff rotas.
Clinical supervision	Clinical supervision provides a safe and confidential environment for you to reflect on practice and discuss issues from work.
	A clinical supervisor is allocated to clinically supervise you individually (a 1:1 clinical supervision approach) or within a clinical supervision group. Your clinical supervisor focuses on support and personal / professional development through the use of reflection.
	Some employers allocate you a local clinical supervisor when you start in practice; others wait for you to request a supervisor, as clinical supervision is self-directed.
	Check whether you are allocated a clinical supervisor automatically or need to contact someone.

(continued)

Table 9.5: (Continued)

Support	Pointers
Action learning sets	Action learning sets facilitated by an experienced nurse are sometimes offered to small groups of nurses to enable them to reflect on specific practice issues.
	One action learning group member presents a specific issue from practice to the group that they wish to take forward with the group's help. The action learning group members support and challenge the nurse through questioning and going through a full action learning cycle (McGill and Beatty, 1992).
National networks / online forums	There are many professional networks and online forums that you can join to keep up to date with the latest initiatives.
	The RCN has a wide range of professional forums and networks that are excellent and free to join.
	Never make a comment on a professional or social media platform which you would not wish to be viewed publicly.
	It is helpful to review the NMC's (2015b) *'Guidance on Using Social Media Responsibly'*.
	Never discuss matters relating to patients outside their clinical area.
Occupational health (OH)	OH departments offer free advice and support linked to keeping staff well. They do not just work with staff that are ill, as they aim to maintain a healthy workforce.
	You can visit your OH department for independent advice on intermittent health problems, lifestyle issues, health promotion and wellbeing services.
Employee assistance programme (EAP)	An EAP is an employee benefit scheme intended to help employees deal with personal problems that might negatively impact their work performance, health or wellbeing.
	An EAP generally includes assessment, counselling and referral services for employees and their immediate family.
Human resources (HR)	HR departments offer advice and support relating to workplace-related issues such as:
	• bullying and harassment
	• disciplinary procedures
	• grievance procedure
	• raising concerns (whistleblowing) policy
	• social media policy
	• workforce equality, diversity and inclusion policy.
	When you start in practice, review the key policies above, as they will clearly set out defined processes for employees to raise issues of concern and access any additional support required.

Table 9.6: QAA credit system

Type of course	Credit level	Total credits
Doctorate (PhD/DPhil)	Level 8	540 credits
Masters	Level 7	480 credits
Degree (BA/BSc)	Level 6	360 credits
Foundation degree	Level 5	240 credits
Apprenticeship	Level 3	120 credits

NOTE: *Credits may vary across certain university courses.*

A number of credits are normally assigned to each module, which indicates the amount of learning undertaken, and credits are awarded once you pass a module. Modules are classed as single or double/treble and the amount of credits awarded align accordingly.

**Credits awarded on 1 × double module =
the credits awarded on 2 × single modules**

Your module credits are accumulated, like building blocks, until you achieve the total credit required for the final academic qualification. You should contact individual universities to establish what the requirements are for any specific programmes you are interested in.

The QAA credit system allows you to accrue credits that may be required on another course, e.g. the first year of a BSc (Hons) degree may be used to transfer to the second year on another degree. Non-UK trained nurses may wish to have previous post-qualification courses accredited from outside the UK. Universities in the UK can use the Accreditation of Prior Experiential Learning (APEL) system which is recognised internationally. The nurse usually requires a transcript from their previous university, an academic statement from a personal tutor for verification, and example work to demonstrate they have covered the module content required to cover the APEL requested.

Time required in notional hours

The amount of learning indicated by a credit value on a module or course is based on the total number of notional hours of learning. The number of notional hours of learning provides a guide as to how long it will take an average student to achieve the module/course outcomes. Within the UK, one credit represents 10 notional hours of learning.

- **150 notional hours of learning on a module will be assigned 15 credits**
- **400 notional hours of learning on a module will be assigned 40 credits**

Accessing funding and study time for post-qualification courses

You may have a clear career plan, but you cannot presume your employer will support a request for time out from practice to attend university every week, or provide financial support to cover your study days or course fees. Accessing post-qualification course funding and paid study time is increasingly competitive.

You can of course self-fund modules, which is what I did to complete a part time BSc (Hons) degree.

When you qualify, your employer will define how many annual paid study and leave days you are entitled to. Managers can allow staff to use their day off or annual leave to attend university if they have no study leave left. However, even if you decide to self-fund, your manager can refuse your request for a set day off to attend university if there is a risk to their service, e.g. you are the only band 5 available to run an outpatient clinic every Monday. Prior to self-funding a course, always check that your manager will support your attendance on a set study day. The alternative to taught study is flexible online or distance learning courses, which are self-directed, and course content can be completed anywhere that suits you.

When applying for course funding, try to understand your manager's perspective, as university fees can cost thousands of pounds for one staff member. If you receive paid study leave this is a further cost implication to their service. When applying for courses, your manager will want to know that you are going to use the course to benefit their service and stay for at least a year after completion. A number of employers request that staff sign a formal contract that includes a clause whereby the individual must pay back a percentage of any funding they received, if they leave their institution within a year or two of completing their course.

If a specialist course is popular, managers usually require a formal application for funding. This entails a shortlisting process, interview and/or presentation. Spend time preparing your application, making sure your personal statement clearly sets out how you will use the course or study time to benefit the practice area that is funding you. You should align previous practice development to your specialist area, ideally demonstrating evidence within your professional portfolio, and show passion and enthusiasm for your current role (see strategies detailed in *Section 9.1*).

REFERENCES

Academy of Medical Royal Colleges (2016) *The Foundation Programme Curriculum: 2016.* London: Academy of Medical Royal Colleges.

Bright, J. (1997) *Turning the Tide.* London: Demos Publishing.

Department of Health (2004) *The NHS Knowledge and Skills Framework (NHS KSF) and the Development Review Process (DH 40440).* London: Stationery Office.

Department of Health, Social Services and Public Safety (2015) *Guidance Notes for Organisations using KSF Development Review/Appraisal to Support Nurses and Midwives with NMC Revalidation (December 2015).* London: DHSSPS.

House of Commons Health Committee (2018) *The Nursing Workforce Second Report of Session 2017–2018.* London: House of Commons Health Committee.

Jackson, D., Firtko, A. and Edenborough, M. (2007) Personal resilience as a strategy for surviving and thriving in the face of workplace adversity: a literature review. *Journal of Advanced Nursing*, 60(1): 1–9.

Kirrane, C. (1993) Informed help wanted on making post-basic education choices. *Nursing Times*, **89**(7): 12.

McGill, I. and Beatty, L. (1992) *Action Learning: a practitioner's guide.* London: Kogan Page.

Nursing and Midwifery Council (2015a) *The Code: professional standards of practice and behaviour for nurses and midwives.* London: NMC.

Nursing and Midwifery Council (2015b) *Guidance on Using Social Media Responsibly.* London: NMC.

Nursing and Midwifery Council (2018a) *Realising Professionalism: Standards for education and training Part 2: standards for student supervision and assessment.* Available at: www.nmc.org.uk/globalassets/sitedocuments/education-standards/student-supervision-assessment.pdf (last accessed 19 July 2018)

Nursing and Midwifery Council (2018b) *Revalidation Resources: forms and templates.* London: NMC.

QAA (2009) *Academic Credit in Higher Education in England – an introduction.* Gloucester: The Quality Assurance Agency for Higher Education.

Royal College of Nursing (2018) *Careers Resources for Nurses and Midwives.* London: RCN.

Willis, P. (2012) *Quality with Compassion: the future of nursing education.* Report of the Willis Commission. London: Royal College of Nursing.

--- **WHAT TO DO NEXT** ---

1. Review opportunities for career progression and align potential roles to professional and academic requirements.

2. Establish what is expected of a band 5 in your area following your preceptorship period.

3. Identify policies and frameworks used by your employer to structure your future professional development reviews and training needs.

4. Familiarise yourself with local appraisal structures in advance for your future appraisals.

5. Start a professional portfolio and begin collecting evidence for revalidation and future funding applications.

6. Check when you are expected to start supervising and assessing students in practice.

7. Find out where you can access additional support to decrease your stress levels and promote resilience to maintain positivity at work.

CHAPTER 10

DEVELOPING OUR PRACTICE AND PROFESSION THROUGH FUTURE NURSING RESEARCH

❝ *Whilst working as a sister, I have never forgotten a conversation I had with a first year student, who said to me:* "It has taken us 45 minutes to hoist Mr X in the bath, shave him, and dress him properly. We have eight patients who need baths this morning, that means it will take us 6 hours just to bathe them all properly without feeding them, doing observations, their risk assessments, pre-op preparation, admissions, meds, toileting and answering buzzers. We only have 8 hours in a shift, so how are we going to fit it all in?" *She looked at me and suddenly the penny dropped ....* "Welcome to nursing", *I said.*

We have more nurses conducting research across the UK than ever before, but we have to question why we have neglected to conduct research examining the fundamentals of nursing care delivered at the bedside, or within a practice clinic/theatre/community setting. How does quality nursing care equate to time spent between a nurse and patient? How long does it take to deliver fundamental nursing care interventions competently? How do quality nurse–patient interactions translate into staffing levels and skill mix? Do untrained : trained nurse staffing ratios influence the standard of care being delivered? We will continue to be told what our minimum nurse staffing levels and staffing ratios should be, until nurses in the future are inspired to conduct observational and quantitative/qualitative research attempting to answer some of these research questions. ❞

Carol Forde-Johnston, lecturer practitioner

I initially contemplated placing this final chapter at the end of another chapter. However, although this is the shortest chapter in this book, its brevity belies the importance of the topic. Future research is central to the development of our profession and promotion of positive change within health care. When I was a student, there were no research or specialist nursing posts to aspire to. Nurses today are trained to question their practice, and nursing curricula equip students with the skills to become research-active. There has never been a time when national research funding has been so accessible to nurses. These opportunities have inevitably increased the number of nurses conducting research in their field, which is remarkable to observe.

Many students and junior nurses I support aspire to become research-active, but workload demands and a lack of protected research time can prevent them from reaching their goals. Barriers can be overcome through funding that enables nurses to have protected study time to conduct research. This chapter presents an overview of how nursing research can influence practice and provides guidance on how to access support for research projects and publish your work in the future.

10.1 EVIDENCE-BASED PRACTICE

During your training, you have been taught to question your practice and critically appraise an evidence base to answer a question. In turn, this enables you to apply the best available evidence to the decisions you make in clinical practice, essentially providing evidence-based practice. The NMC (2015) *Code* requires nurses to *'deliver care based on the best available evidence or best practice'* and you have been trained to acquire evidence from appropriate local and national intranet sites and databases. The new NMC (2018) standards of proficiency for registered nurses call for registered nurses to provide evidence-based nursing care in the future, *'using best-practice approaches'* across many clinical skills relating to proficiencies and procedural competencies.

In 1991, the Department of Health introduced the first national research strategy to provide a coordinated approach to promoting evidence-based practice (DH, 1991). National initiatives were subsequently launched, including:

- the **NHS Centre for Reviews and Dissemination** (NHS CRD): the NHS CRD provides the NHS with information on the effectiveness of treatments. It is a world renowned organisation that produces policy-relevant research aiming to promote research evidence that improves health.

- the National Institute for Health and Care Excellence (NICE): NICE is an NHS agency that promotes clinical excellence and cost-effectiveness. NICE develops guidance and recommendations on the effectiveness of treatments and medical procedures.

Since the early 1990s, these institutions have continued to thrive and are important disseminators of up-to-date guidelines and recommendations for health care professionals. Nowadays, we also have the Cochrane library:

- The Cochrane library provides free online access to high quality systematic reviews in over 100 countries. The library organises medical findings, which inform evidence-based choices about health interventions.

If you work for the NHS make sure you join your local NHS health care library, to register with an NHS account and access free NHS Athens electronic resources.

Find an area of interest you are passionate about

Some of the most influential research has been prompted simply by a hunch, an initial spark of interest, a particular event or anecdotal evidence. I remember working in a neurology unit in the 1980s as a student. It was widely recognised by doctors and nurses at the time that patients were regularly smoking marijuana to control muscle spasms associated with multiple sclerosis. I remember a very strict matron turning a blind eye when patients brought marijuana in, as long as they did not smoke on hospital premises and they kept it locked up (considered completely unacceptable nowadays). It was largely due to anecdotal evidence and charitable support from the MS Society that, years later, national research trials were conducted. Today medicinal cannabis is offered as a standard treatment in the form of Sativex, which is specifically licensed to treat muscle spasms and stiffness in MS.

In 2017, a lady called Joy Milne was reported across UK media outlets as being able to *"smell her husband's Parkinson's disease"*. The lady in question had recently joined the charity Parkinson's UK and informed a doctor at the meeting about this oddity. The doctor decided to examine this anomaly further and Ms Milne was asked to attend a pilot study. She correctly identified which seven people, from a group of 24, had Parkinson's disease, by sniffing T-shirts they had worn for a day. Parkinson's UK is currently funding a collaborative research study with the Universities of Manchester and Edinburgh to identify the molecules in sebum that cause the odour. If successful, a potential diagnostic tool may be created in the future. It is amazing that this interesting study snowballed from a passing conversation and a hunch and that, as a result, individuals around the world may be diagnosed with Parkinson's disease more quickly.

The most inspiring researchers I have worked with have been totally absorbed in their subject and passionate about influencing practice through networking. I meet many nurses who have a fantastic researchable area but are put off by the academia surrounding research, or they do not think they have the skills to conduct research, or write it up afterwards. Try to think positively and do not give up; if you are passionate about an area, others will be too. Speak to related charitable organisations and network with experts in the field. Many NHS employers are supporting staff to become active researchers through education, research training groups and regular research networking events.

The importance of research within our profession

Documented nursing research was first carried out by Florence Nightingale, and her passion for statistics gave her a sound evidence base to argue for improved sanitation. She used survey instruments, graphical data and pie charts to disseminate her research findings, such as high mortality rates relating to *'certain conditions'* (Nightingale, 1859). Florence Nightingale was the first nurse researcher to compare mortality rates associated with care delivered by trained versus untrained nurses. These findings enabled her to acquire financial support to establish the first training school for nurses at St Thomas' Hospital, London (Nightingale, 1863).

Two other nursing pioneers, Dr Nancy Bergstrom and Barbara Braden, collaboratively developed and tested the Braden scale for predicting pressure sore risk, which is used worldwide by nurses in practice today (Bergstrom *et al.*, 1996). Florence Nightingale, Barbara Braden and Nancy Bergstrom were nursing innovators and their research studies have commonalities. They created an evidence base that included large amounts of quantitative data, they networked and collaborated with relevant others to support their study, they chose research areas that had relevance for patients and their study findings clearly impacted on patient outcomes.

Qualitative versus quantitative research

Over my nursing career, I have noted that there has always been an undercurrent of two camps of research and evidence in health care, between nursing and medical professional groups. In simplistic terms, nursing research has tended to be more qualitative and evaluative, as nurses talk and use words to care. In contrast, medics prescribe interventions and use quantitative research that includes statistics, randomised controlled trials and double-blind studies. You can observe these unsophisticated descriptions when comparing most nursing and medical journals.

The tide is changing, however, as more nursing researchers are including quantitative approaches or mixed method research designs within their studies, providing hard evidence for change. NHS CRD, NICE and the Cochrane Database of Systematic Reviews are full of medical research, as scientific research approaches are deemed to be more reliable by government and public bodies. Randomised controlled trials and double-blind trials reduce bias, and are considered the most reliable form of primary research in the field of health interventions.

There is great value in good qualitative research used in the right context for the right research question. However, we also need a quantitative evidence base to inform the delivery of fundamental nursing interventions and the examination of nurse–patient interactions. Government departments and policy makers are not going to increase nursing staff levels with more qualitative staff surveys, telling us how nurses feel and what they experience at work.

The argument against quantifying the art of nursing is that the dynamic nature of nursing cannot be captured numerically. I agree that human nuances of caring, empathy and compassion do not fit with numerical values and need to be described or experienced. However, ignoring the scientific aspects of nursing interventions being delivered has left us with a lack of hard evidence to justify the time we need to spend with our patients delivering quality care. Determining **average unit times** for key nursing interventions in hospital and community settings through national observational, comparative and experimental research studies would inform the gap in the current evidence base. Average unit times could be aligned with low, medium or high patient acuity and dependency scores.

What is the average time to competently and safely deliver key inpatient hospital interventions? For example, the time taken to:

- carry out a full bed bath that includes an individual's full hygiene needs, hair, oral care, etc. (can be multiplied according to number of patients requiring baths on a shift)

- administer one oral tablet or IV (includes checking patient and preparation through to discarding sharps; can be multiplied according to prescribed medications)

- document each of the national patient risk assessments and implement and evaluate strategies in place to prevent risks

- use manual handling aids to transfer patients in/out of bed

- complete a set of vital signs and escalation pathways

- feed a meal to a patient who cannot feed themselves

- complete a comprehensive mental capacity assessment

- communicate with an individual to complete an holistic assessment on admission

- conduct a safe discharge or nursing transfer for a patient

- assess and dress wounds of different grades.

The power of nursing research cannot be underestimated, and there will always be a place for both qualitative and quantitative nursing research. However, the first question most clinicians are asked if they want to innovate or initiate a change, or ask for more staff, is *"Where is your evidence?"*, with the word evidence usually being a synonym for statistics and numbers in today's health care. Surely, more quantitative data relating to nursing interventions has the potential to better inform current patient dependency and acuity tools, safe staffing tools and care hours required. In summary, nursing research is important to the future of our profession and it needs to be the right kind of research to answer the right questions.

10.2 RESEARCH FUNDING OPPORTUNITIES

If you are interested in pursuing a career in research you can align your experiences and professional achievements to a research career pathway (see *Table 9.1*). There are many types of post you can apply for that will include active involvement on funded research projects, such as a university nurse educator, research nurse, advanced nurse practitioner and specialist nurse. If research is an inherent part of your role, you should aim to publish in collaboration with the research team you are working with.

External funding streams can support innovative ideas for research projects and cover staff time out, e.g. a paid research study day every week for a year. Many charitable organisations also provide research funding opportunities that health care professionals can apply for. As a self-funding PhD student, I have managed to secure funding for my course fees every year from a wide range of charitable organisations. It took many hours to complete the funding applications, but the effort was worth every hour spent.

Where do I apply for research funding?

If your current role does not allow you time to conduct active research, start by asking your employer whether they would allocate you protected research time in the future. You will need to discuss your ideas with your line manager and have a thorough research plan/proposal prepared, which is written and summarised succinctly.

Aim to align your research project to the goals of the organisation you work for, and clearly outline how improvements can be informed by your research. There are experienced researchers available to help guide your preparation, whom you can contact online through local research departments and the National Institute for Health Research (NIHR).

Nurses who successfully achieve employer support do not just have a chat about their idea to their manager. They present an informed argument by contacting other units and researchers in the field to scope what is happening nationally. They also network with local teams, medics or AHPs, present a literature review and summary of the current evidence base, and identify potential benefits/cost savings to patient services.

If your manager is unable to support protected research study, do not give up – try to find alternative funding. There are two main national funding streams you can target: **government funding** and **charitable funding**. Some examples of funding streams and guidance are presented in *Table 10.1*.

Table 10.1: Some examples of where to apply for research funding

Institution	Awards
Health Education England (HEE) and the National Institute for Health Research (NIHR)	**Pre-doctoral clinical academic fellowships:** these enable staff to split their time equally between clinical service and academic training over a 2-year period through protected time. These fellowships and awards are very competitive and there is clear guidance on websites for applicants.
	Training and career development awards: funding up to £5500, for any nurse or AHP engaged in research for a short course or modules, which provide training and expertise in research skills or research management.
Local research committees	**Oxfordshire Health Research Committee small grants:** check your local employer and regional research grants. Within my local region of Oxfordshire, grants of up to £10 000 have been offered to salaried staff working within the NHS in Oxfordshire.
RCN foundation bursary schemes	**Bursaries:** professional bursaries of up to £5000 available for career development activities, which focus on primary care or long-term conditions, e.g. obesity, mental health, children's/young people's services, older people and dementia. These awards are also open to health care assistants and assistant practitioners.
UK charities	**Funding for research studies aligned to the charity patient group:** funding can include conducting a study, paid time out and funding for research equipment costs. Online application criteria will be set by the charity and your study outcomes must focus on the related patient group, e.g. Parkinson's UK.

10.3 PUBLISHING YOUR WORK IN THE FUTURE

Despite increasing numbers of nurses with degrees and Masters within our profession, only a small proportion seek to publish their work. As a profession we need to question why this is the case and put strategies in place to promote nurses' publishing. When I am trying to encourage qualified staff or students to publish, they often think that their project is not interesting enough or they do not have the writing standard required. NHS employers and universities aim to encourage staff and students to publish, but there is a need to offer study time and regular writing/publication workshops. Practice supervisors and assessors who have published could potentially guide those who wish to publish, and more collaborative publications should be encouraged.

Remember that published work does not have to be an in-depth research study or systematic review. I started with a letter in the *Nursing Times* when I had just qualified. Just sharing your perspectives and experiences can be relevant to a topical area and interesting for others to read. Writing up a service evaluation or a change you have implemented in practice can inform readers who may be dealing with a similar practice situation. If you have something interesting to say, try to put pen to paper, as your voice is just as worthy as anyone else's!

Evidence of published work is very good to have on your CV when you apply for jobs or courses. Publications show that you are motivated and passionate about a specialist field and can set you apart from other candidates. I offer workshops to staff and students, to encourage them to publish, and have presented a few tips to motivate and guide you (see *Table 10.2*).

Table 10.2: Tips to help you publish your work

Tips	Further guidance
Start with an area of interest	Thought-provoking publications are written by someone who is passionate about a topic, has experiences to share or can present a fresh approach to a relevant subject.
	• Could you write up a recent literature review or summarise recommendations from an assignment?
	• Could you share or compare personal experiences, e.g. the transition from being a student to qualified?
	• Are you interested in piloting something new in practice, which could be written up as an evaluative project?
	• Have you conducted a research study, which could be summarised for an article?
Choose the right type of article	Decide which type of article suits your content, e.g. literature review, systematic review, original research or innovations in practice, such as service evaluations.
	Online journal guidance will indicate which type of article suits your work.
Choose the right journal	Journals may have a variety of styles, as they have different target audiences.
	Establish which journals best suit your style by reading a selection of articles from a number of journals.

(continued)

Table 10.2: (Continued)

Tips	Further guidance
Download author guides	Every journal will have an *'Author guide'* that you can download from their website.
	Always adhere to this author guidance, e.g. keep within word limit, use Harvard referencing and the correct headings / font size.
	Always proofread! An editor reads thousands of papers and will not spend time correcting your work. Many papers are rejected at an early stage, due to a lack of proofreading or adherence to journal guidance.
Contact editors	Contact editors about your topic before you send any papers to them for review. This will enable you to find out whether or not they are actually interested in publishing your work. A quick email or phone call will establish whether an editor is interested.
	Once you submit a paper for review it can take many weeks for a response. During this time it is unethical to submit your paper elsewhere. If you have submitted your paper to an editor who has already covered your topic a few months ago, you may waste time waiting for their rejection.
	Editors are usually very honest and helpful. If they reject your topic they often advise alternative journals and offer constructive suggestions to improve your paper.
Start simple and use headings	Start off with a smaller piece of writing, e.g. write a letter, case study or reflective piece.
	Start an article, or chapter, with key headings first. It is much easier to motivate yourself to write, and less daunting, when you are faced with writing a page or two for one section.
Attend workshops and writing groups	Attend writing and publication workshops / study days that are available at local or national level.
	Writing groups help to motivate writers, as time is set aside to write during the event.
	Many large NHS employers have researcher coffee mornings and networking groups. These are helpful if you wish to collaborate with others on projects or publications. NHS research departments send out global emails advertising these events and you will need to sign up to receive regular updates.
Collaborate with a co-author	If you find writing for publication especially challenging, try collaborating with a co-author.
	If you have difficulties finding a co-author ask local universities, as they aim to promote publications across all fields.

REFERENCES

Bergstrom, N., Braden, B., Kemp, M. *et al.* (1996) Multi-site study of incidence of pressure ulcers and the relationship between risk level, demographic characteristics, diagnoses, and prescription of preventive interventions. *Journal of the American Geriatrics Society*, **44**(1): 22–30.

Department of Health (1991) *Research for Health: a research and development strategy for the NHS*. London: HMSO.

Nightingale, F. (1859) *A Contribution to the Sanitary History of the British Army During the Late War with Russia*. London: John W. Parker and Sons.

Nightingale, F. (1863) *Notes on Hospitals*. London: Longman, Green, Roberts, and Green.

Nursing and Midwifery Council (2015) *The Code: professional standards of practice and behaviour for nurses and midwives*. London: NMC.

Nursing and Midwifery Council (2018) *Future Nurse: standards of proficiency for registered nurses*. Available at: www.nmc.org.uk/globalassets/sitedocuments/education-standards/future-nurse-proficiencies.pdf (last accessed 19 July 2018)

—————————— WHAT TO DO NEXT ——————————

1. Contact senior researchers and educators locally to identify opportunities for conducting research and publishing in your current role, and discuss potential ideas with a research-active experienced nurse.

2. Join local clinical research groups to discuss your area of interest and network with like-minded colleagues.

3. Attend local and national publishing workshops or complete online 'how to publish' programmes.

4. Contact the local university health care department to identify any collaborative research projects you could help support.

5. Review local and national funding streams and the deadlines for funding applications. This may enable you to have paid time out or pay for future course fees.

INDEX